# The GOOD SLIMMING GUIDE

*HOW TO CHOOSE
THE DIET OR TREATMENT
THAT'S BEST FOR YOU*

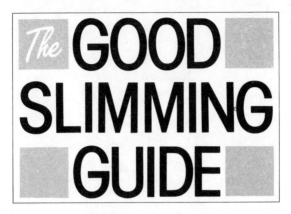

# The GOOD SLIMMING GUIDE

### *HOW TO CHOOSE*
### *THE DIET OR TREATMENT*
### *THAT'S BEST FOR YOU*

## ALIX KIRSTA

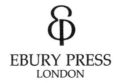

EBURY PRESS
LONDON

Published by Ebury Press
Division of The National Magazine Company Ltd
Colquhoun House
27–37 Broadwick Street
London   W1V 1FR

First Impression 1987
Text copyright © 1987 by Alix Kirsta

ISBN 0 85223 660 3

Editor: Suzanne Webber
Designer: Roger Daniels

Computerset by MFK Typesetting Ltd, Hitchin, Herts

Printed and bound in Great Britain at The Bath Press,
Bath, Avon

# Contents

# *Introduction*

You take off your clothes. You stand in front of the mirror. You then take a long critical look at your body. Now for that moment of truth. How pleased are you with what you see? Probably not entirely, perhaps not at all. Is there room for improvement? If you're truthful, almost certainly. This may involve only very subtle and miniscule modifications, or a major body rethink.

Throughout the country millions of women, and probably a fair proportion of men, go through this salutary ritual of self-evaluation, notching up pluses and minuses against their physical appearance. More often than not, points against will outnumber points in favour. Few of us would claim, even at the best of times, to be completely satisfied with the way nature has assembled the raw materials that make up our physique.

Weight problems, however, are always relative, overweight inevitably a matter of degree. Take the woman who can no longer get into her figure-hugging jeans and dresses because she has put on an extra seven pounds (3 kg): her drive to slim may be as strong as that of someone struggling to drop from 15 stone (210 lbs/95 kg) to 11 (154 lbs/70 kg). The approach adopted by two such people to cope with these very different problems will, however, vary enormously. It will be coloured by varying individual attitudes to body image, lifestyle, food and eating.

That is basically what this book is all about – evaluating the relative merits of different popular diets and treatments. The aim is to get a clearer picture of the various options available to anyone embarking on the often confusing and frustrating business of shaping up and shedding weight. Finding a 'best way' to slim becomes more perplexing with each passing year. There has surely never been such a formidable choice of diets, products, treatments and supplements.

## SLIMMER'S CHOICES
### WHAT'S THE BEST WAY FOR YOU?

Slimmers are often grouped together by slimming magazines or slimming product manufacturers regardless of whether the slimmer has just a few pounds (kilos) to lose to get into a special outfit, or a long-term more serious weight problem, perhaps linked to stress. This chart will help you to find the diets or treatments that will be best for your particular problems. Find the problem that most closely matches your own case, and read the relevant sections of the book for a detailed description of the type of diets or treatments recommended. Your choice will then be much easier.

Before tackling any weight problem it is important to recognise your basic body type. The three types are: endomorph, mesomorph and ectomorph. Each has distinctive features.

| | |
|---|---|
| *Endomorph* | Generally heavy in build and relatively shortlimbed. |
| *Mesomorph* | Innately muscular in body structure. |
| *Ectomorph* | Lean-bodied. |

## PROBLEM

Typical Endomorph – body type predisposed to weight gain. Longterm problem of excessive overweight, 5 (70 lbs/31 kg) or 6 stone (84 lbs/38 kg). Sedentary lifestyle, inability to stick to a reducing diet.

## METHOD

Join a slimming group (see pp 127–129) such as Weight Watchers for support, encouragement and advice on a healthy, non fattening diet as opposed to a very restricted regime. In addition, take up regular, initially not too vigorous, exercise (see pp 95–115) such as fast walking, swimming, keep fit classes or join a health club to boost morale and motivation. This is the time to experiment with a new, non fattening but balanced diet to last you for life. Try F-Plan diet (see p 40).

## PROBLEM

About 1–1½ stone (14–21 lbs/6–9 kg) overweight gained over 18 months due to stress, 'comfort' eating in response to loneliness, depression and inactivity. Half-hearted, failed attempts at dieting, followed by rebound 'bingeing'.

## METHOD

Join a slimming club or group therapy (see pp 127–129) in order to try and work out underlying emotional problems behind erratic eating habits. Join a sports club, take up exercising with a friend for company and support (see p 99). You should stick to a balanced diet to maintain energy. Base this on high-fibre, high complex-carbohydrate foods as in F-Plan or Pritikin diets (see pp 40 and 36).

## PROBLEM

Typical Mesomorph – greater ratio of muscle to fat makes for stocky build which can turn to fat with decreased physical activity/increased food intake. About 1 stone (14 lbs/6 kg) overweight, gained rapidly through increasingly sedentary, 'middle-aged' lifestyle, diet high in sweet, fatty foods, increased alcohol consumption. Attempts to modify this have failed over longer periods and weight is increasing.

## METHOD

Try a rapid weight-loss diet for fast, visible results. This should provide an incentive to then modify long-term eating habits. Best bets – Scarsdale Diet (see p. 32), Cambridge or similar VLCD (see p 47), Beverly Hills Diet (see p 42). Then switch to sensible eating plan, low fat, high complex carbohydrate (see p 15). Limit alcohol to one or two glasses of wine per week. Cut out all sweets, fried and fatty foods. Take up regular vigorous aerobic exercise to help rev up metabolism (see pp 103–105).

## PROBLEM

Typical Ectomorph, the type that's normally very slim, especially in youth, and sleekly proportioned, as long as metabolism allows rapid, efficient burn up of Calories (kilojoules). This mechanism can slow down with age, so now only 4 to 6 lbs (2–3 kg) overweight, but reflected in a typical 'pear shape', excess fat concentrated on hips and thighs.

## METHOD

Maintain a well balanced, varied diet, low in fats and sweet foods. It should be relatively salt-free to counteract fluid retention, which can aggravate tendency towards pear shape. Drink plenty of water or herbal infusions to act as mild diuretic. Follow regular exercise programme – gym or Pilates workout (see p 111) to tighten specific areas. Alternate with swimming and/or dance or keep fit classes (see p 105) to trim lower half of body and tighten muscles. Intensive course of CTM or vacuum suction massage (see pp 75–78) or Mesotherapy micro-injections to boost circulation and redistribute hardened fat on hips and thighs (see p 83–84).

## PROBLEM

Weight normal or near normal but very pronounced imbalance of lower and upper body due to build up of fatty tissue on bottom and thighs and underdeveloped upper body (inherited body type).

## METHOD

Regular exercise, swimming, dancing, gym (preferably Hydra-fitness), Pilates, to build upper body, tighten and elongate muscles of legs, flatten buttocks (see p 111). Very extreme measure, surgical liposuction to remove excess fat if skin is resilient (see p 139).

## PROBLEM

Near normal weight but flabby, slack tummy muscles.

## METHOD

Begin with a course of Slendertone passive slimming treatments (see p 90) if very unfit, especially after pregnancy, then graduate to regular exercise programme (see p 99) – dance, keep fit classes, gym workouts with emphasis on sit-ups to tighten tummy muscles. Extreme measure to counteract loose stomach tissues – a surgical 'tummy tuck' (see p 135).

### PROBLEM

A long-term, persistent weight problem, 1½ stone (21 lbs/9 kg) overweight in spite of very physically active lifestyle. Constant hunger, tendency to expend a lot of energy, persistent faintness and tiredness when on a Calorie (kilojoule) restricted diet makes weight reduction a near impossibility.

### METHOD

Cut down gradually on 'fast energy' comfort foods such as chocolate, buns, biscuits, fried fatty food. Replace these with wholegrains, pulses, vegetables, fruit, cereals, which release energy slowly and keep blood sugar consistently high for long periods. Try auriculotherapy or regular acupuncture (see p 117) to combat hunger pangs and cravings for sweet food. Hypnosis may also solve this problem (see p 124). If energy is extra low before or during bouts of exercise or intensive activity, take a balanced formula meal replacement drink or crunchy bar to boost energy – i.e. Cambridge (see p 47).

### PROBLEM

Typical middle-aged male figure/weight problem: 2½ stone (35 lbs/16 kg) overweight gained over five years due to increased alcohol intake, entertaining (business lunches, travel, etc.) coupled with less active lifestyle. Fat most noticeable around stomach – typical 'pot belly'.

### METHOD

Limit alcohol to wine only or wine and mineral water mix. Cut out beer altogether. Eliminate or ration spirits. Cut down drastically on fats i.e. butter, eggs, cheese, milk, red meat, sausages, bacon and all rich, sweet foods. Increase intake of low Calorie (kilojoule), complex carbohydrates (see p 15). To help adhere to new healthy pattern of eating go on Scarsdale Diet (see p 32) or F-Plan Diet (see p 40) for rapid results. Take up regular vigorous exercise programme, concentrating on aerobic activities to strengthen and protect cardiovascular system and lungs while boosting metabolism. Gym workouts will tighten stomach muscles (see p 108).

**The media and the message**

The quest for perfect, or as near perfect as possible, physical proportions has spawned a burgeoning industry. This industry is devoted exclusively to helping men and women of all shapes and sizes attain today's streamlined, lean and taut-limbed ideal. In Europe and America slimming has become a major preoccupation, sometimes bordering on obsession. The criteria by which we judge physical aesthetics are today narrower and more strictly defined than at any other time in history. The fashions we wear, the lifestyles we pursue nowadays allow little opportunity to camouflage shortcomings. We cannot comfortably get away with any major deviation from the established norm. Like it or not, a slim, firm, fit and well-proportioned body, male or female, represents today's physical ideal. It embodies the quintessence of youth and sexual attractiveness, exuding fitness and good health.

Whether subliminal or overt, the message propounded by the media and advertising industry alike is inescapably clear. To be overweight is undesirable and unattractive, while to be super-slim is sexy, fashionable and desirable. It is hardly surprising that someone with even a minor figure problem may develop a complex inappropriate and out of proportion to the actual problem.

But then body image, if we're honest about it, linked as it is to sexuality and self-esteem is a highly emotive issue for most of us. It is surely because of this that common sense, objectivity and logic often lose out to hope, credulity and desperation. Women in particular aspire to what sometimes seem to be almost unattainably high standards of physical perfection.

**Raising our health consciousness**

Yet vanity, fashion consciousness and a concern for self image are not the sole factors that motivate the majority of people to slim. The phenomenal, ever expanding growth in health consciousness has developed over just a few years. It has led increasing numbers of men and women to revolutionise their attitudes to diet, exercise, stress, and weight gain. It has meant that most of us are now intent on controlling or reducing weight, not just in order to look good, but to feel healthier. In just a few years weight control has gone from being a beauty problem to a health issue.

This concern for improving health is far from misplaced. Weight problems, ranging from the transitory and minimal to the chronic and life-threatening, are no longer the exception but increasingly the rule in industrialised society. The disturbing fact is that obesity is fast becoming a national malady, yet one which is almost certainly largely self-generated.

In terms of staying healthy, most attempts to lose weight or avoid getting fat in the first place are therefore totally justified. The statistics concerning fat people are certainly scary, and the health hazards of being fat have been unequivocally hammered home by the medical profession. By now they make familiar reading. The more overweight you are, the higher the risk you run of developing diseases such as diabetes, hypertension, cardiovascular disease, respiratory disorders. Circulatory ailments, arthritis and other aches and pains of the joints are also frequently aggravated by the physical strain of carrying around too much extra weight. Complications during pregnancy are also far more common amongst women who are overweight and who gain weight excessively while they are pregnant. Grossly overweight people are also likely to die at an earlier age than those of normal weight. Being slim is not merely fashionable and sexy; more important, it is healthy.

### Why we're getting fatter

But why is it that we are becoming fatter? Apart from those cases where excess weight is linked to a metabolic defect or serious illness, current evidence points to lifestyle. In particular our eating habits are cited as the prime culprit of weight gain. The tendency to gain weight sometimes runs in families. Body type, too, which predisposes certain people to gain weight more easily than others can prove an inbuilt handicap for those engaged in a battle against bulge and flab. But while it is certainly tempting to blame your genes or glands for being overweight, it is also usually misguided and inaccurate. The majority of us who are overweight are so mainly through eating too much while exercising too little. It is a simple example of too much energy input, too little energy output, resulting in an energy surplus: one of the basic laws of thermodynamics!

**Why the slim want to be slimmer**
Paradoxically, slimming is not an activity confined merely to those people who are overweight. Far from it. Many apparently slim women and girls become analytical about their bodies, to the point of near neurosis. Even 'slim' people are concerned about body image. The desire to look as youthful and modish as possible may be coupled with involvement in one of the so-called 'glamour' professions where looks rate high. Or it may be motivated by certain sports where body weight can determine achievement.

Countless women of normal, or even below-normal, weight extend the ranks of those battling with genuine superfluous fat. Their aim is to tighten and trim those parts of the body that do not measure up to total perfection. It is this emphasis on perfect contours and proportion, rather than ideal weight, that now motivates increasing numbers of women to attend exercise classes, gyms and health clubs. Or they pay out vast sums of money on salon treatments for specific 'localised' figure problems. They will even undergo cosmetic surgery to eliminate defects such as cellulite or a flabby tummy.

## Weight to volume

This highlights one essential distinction that divides slimmers into two camps: those concerned with weight, versus those preoccupied with volume. Those trying to 'shape up' as against those wishing mainly to get their weight down. As many dieters know only too well, relying on the scales to spell out your figure problem is often misleading. Most of us care more about what our bodies look like.

The actual distribution of fat, the balance of curves and symmetry of contours, matters more than their sum total in weight. There can, after all, be a tremendous discrepancy between how you measure up and what you weigh. This is why many dieters often remain disappointed with their shape, long after reaching their target weight.

Being of normal or near normal weight, according to height and build, does not necessarily mean your shape is all you'd ideally wish it to be. The scales cannot tell you if you're flabby. Nor can they locate exactly where those last few stubborn pounds (kilos) are lodged as extra inches (centimetres). This is why attempting to slim down specific areas, for example hips and thighs – the notorious female 'pear shape', can prove more difficult than simply trying to reduce overall weight. It is a maddening quirk of sod's law that even after having dieted to reach her lowest possible weight, a typically pear-shaped woman may not look all that different, because of the uneven distribution of fat. That is where exercise comes in. Exercise can sometimes improve body contours quite specifically, to a degree that dieting often fails to do.

## No universal answer

The differing needs, expectations and ultimate goals of body shaping are what make the whole business of slimming such a hit or miss affair for many of us. There is not one single, foolproof method of slimming guaranteed to suit everyone.

Nor could there ever be such a one-for-all system. Any diet or slimming programme, to be universally appealing and successful, would have to fit the vast spectrum of ages, personalities, lifestyles, expectations and priorities of the myriad individuals who make up the 'slimming market'.

What is obvious, however, is that the more tailored your slimming programme to fit in with your life and yourself the more likely it is to help you achieve your aims. Embarking on say, a faddy one-food-only diet if you have to entertain a lot because of your job is clearly a venture doomed to failure. The same is true of a spartan 350-Calorie-a-day (83-kilojoule) regime of meal replacement drinks for a very active person who perpetually suffers hunger pangs and enjoys the ritual of sitting down to meals.

**Eat well, stay slim**

Luckily there is plenty of new research to indicate that you do not have to starve stoically for long periods in order to shed weight. Doctors and dietitians are unanimous about the tremendous advantages of following a diet based mainly on fibre rich, complex-carbohydrate foods such as wholegrains, cereals, pulses, vegetables, fruit and low-fat dairy produce in reducing and regulating weight. These wholefoods should ideally feature as staple, everyday items on any healthy well-balanced diet. If you consciously opt for a low fat, high fibre diet, you are less likely to become fat in the first place.

The current medical verdict is that to protect our health and avoid disease we should drastically limit the amount of sugar, sweet foods, animal protein and saturated fats in our diet. These are all high Calorie (kilojoule) foods which, if eaten to excess will cause the majority of people to gain weight fast and easily. It follows that Calorie controlled eating is something we should undertake for life – not just while slimming.

Better news still, complex-carbohydrate foods go further as

a source of energy. They assuage hunger for longer periods because, unlike fat and sugar which are converted instantly into energy with any unused surplus stored as fat, they are metabolised more slowly and efficiently by the body. Another point to remember about slimming is that the diet most resembling your own established eating habits is the one you are most likely to stick with. This is the diet which will help you lose weight most effectively, and it explains the limited value of gimmicky, fad diets. Aiming for subtle variations and specific restrictions within the framework of a varied, interesting eating plan offers a more realistic chance of slimming successfully than subsisting on lettuce and grapefruit.

**No crash diets**
Another trick to succeeding where so many others fail is to pursue your goals slowly and systematically, avoiding the urge to obtain instant results. The older you are, the more this rule applies. Our base metabolic rate, which keeps bodily functions ticking over, decreases steadily with age. Weight gained in middle age, say from one's thirties or forties onward, is fiendishly difficult to lose, especially if weight gain is accompanied by decreased physical activity.

The psychological motivation that prompts one to overeat is often caused by factors such as stress, depression, loneliness and boredom. It may become more prevalent and less easy to overcome instantly, at will, as we get older. What is more, unhealthy eating habits, for example 'bingeing' or comfort eating, once ingrained, are hard to change without a concerted effort, limitless patience and immense will-power.

The more weight you want to lose, the more time you should be prepared to give yourself for the task. What so many people forget is that the longer the period over which that excess has accumulated, the slower the rate at which it will diminish. Extra weight that creeps up slowly over a few years is far harder to shift permanently than even a stone (14 lbs/ 6 kg) gained rapidly through obvious over-indulgence. The inevitable corollary to this is that weight lost rapidly returns quite rapidly, while weight lost slowly tends to stay off.

Slimming can become an extremely stressful occupation for many people. This is especially so for those who believe, mistakenly, that the only way to achieve their objective is by slavishly following a set of rigid rules and restrictions which any non-slimmer would dismiss as a living nightmare. When it comes to the nitty gritty, it seems to me that sensible, agony-free slimming is as much a matter of reviewing, and where necessary modifying one's lifestyle and behaviour, especially where this involves eating and physical activity, as being clued up about Calories (kilojoules). Developing a clear-minded objectivity, rather than nurturing a hang-up about a particular figure or weight problem makes for relatively stress-free slimming. It allows you to follow those strategies best suited to solving your own individual problem.

**What suits you best**
In the following chapters I have tried to give the low-down on as many different methods and theories of weight loss as possible, as well as providing a review of the currently popular diets and products on the slimming market. Evaluation of these diverse aspects of the industry is at best an arbitrary exercise. Subjective proof and anecdotal evidence, not scientific data, are all I, as a reporter, have to go on in assessing the relative merits of any diet, product or system.

Just because one specific diet, exercise system or therapy works for one person does not mean it will do so for another.

The important thing to bear in mind when shopping around for any 'best bet' to help you slim is that the weight loss business, like the beauty industry to which it is closely allied, addresses itself largely to our hopes and irrational expectations, trading in hollow promises and dreams. Each new slimming craze or dietary fad comes and goes with alarming yet predictable regularity, some worthwhile, others less so. Some demand a suspension of disbelief, others appeal to our better judgement.

I have tried to be fair by reviewing the slimming business as comprehensively as possible, omitting only out and out crank crazes and gimmickry. Above all, I realise that every would-be slimmer has different goals in mind and different ways of realising those goals based on inherent likes and dislikes. My aim in the following chapters is to be both as constructive and as positive as possible when explaining how, why or for whom this or that method may or may not prove helpful.

I have broadened the term 'slimming' to encompass a variety of figure defects and flaws. Any of these might prevent a woman from measuring up to her own physical ideal, or from fulfilling her potential.

Above all, the idea is to dispel some of the myths associated with weight reduction and body shaping while avoiding a dogmatic, doctrinaire approach to the 'best way' of slimming. Trial and error, personal experiment may be your best way of finding out ultimately what suits you and brings results (see chart on pp 8–10 for quick reference).

Lastly, a word of caution. Although this book is written mainly for men and women with varying degrees of weight problems, it is *not* aimed at those who are chronically and severely overweight, or suffering from life-threatening obesity. Anyone with such a condition must consult their doctor in order to determine whether their weight is related to ill-health or glandular dysfunction. These cases require medical treatment. For many people with a severe weight problem, medical treatment is the only way to overcome and control it. Your doctor is the person best qualified to refer you to a clinic specialising in obesity if necessary.

# – 1 –

# *Dieting: Gain or Loss*

An effective weight-reducing diet inevitably forms the cornerstone of any slimming programme. It is virtually impossible for a normal, healthy person to lose a significant amount of weight, except by altering the basic ratio of Calorie (kilojoule) input versus Calorie (kilojoule) output. Weight gain inevitably results when the amount of Calories (kilojoules) provided by the food we eat exceeds the number of Calories (kilojoules) burnt through physical activity and the body's metabolic processes. Although normal body size, skeletal frame and the distribution of fatty tissue are all inherited characteristics (sometimes affected by illness and hormonal defects), it is one of the most demonstrable laws of cause and effect that extra Calories (kilojoules), if not used up in exercise or daily activity, eventually get stored away in the form of superfluous body fat.

### Fluctuating weight

Over the years a person's normal or ideal weight may fluctuate and rise as a result of a gradual lowering of the body's metabolic rate. This lowering begins somewhere between the ages of 35 and 40. Add to this slowing-down process the tendency to take less physical exercise, while perhaps eating more fattening foods, and the results, in terms of an inexorable increase in weight, and visible build-up of superfluous layers of fat, become self-evident.

Degrees of excess weight differ enormously from person to person. They may range from four or seven pounds (2–3 kg) gained, perhaps, quite quickly over a period of obvious over-indulgence – during Christmas or Thanksgiving festivities or a long cold winter, to the two, three or more stones (28–42 lbs/ 12–18 kg) representative of a problem verging on obesity. The strategies for overcoming one person's problem may prove woefully inadequate, or else overly stringent, when applied to someone else's.

Obviously, those with a chronic long-term weight problem, and a natural tendency to gain large amounts of weight, will need to restrict their Calories (kilojoules) intake and make a serious attempt to change their eating habits for a long period, if not for life, if they are seriously committed to becoming slim. The more stubborn the weight problem, the tougher the measures needed to overcome it. There are no instant or easy solutions when it comes to shedding large amounts of excess fat and, more significantly, maintaining that weight-loss.

By comparison, those who are only a few pounds (kilos) overweight may have a relatively easy time trying to slim. They may succeed in doing so by following a few dietary restrictions. They may, for instance, give up sweet foods and sugar in tea and coffee, cutting out potatoes and biscuits or cookies from the daily diet, limiting alcohol intake or doing without that chocolate or candy snack at teatime or the mid-morning break. Easier said than done, however, as with all matters involving self-discipline the fact that the number of lapsed dieters greatly outnumbers the successful ones, testifies to the extremely arduous business of trying to lose weight.

**High drop-out rate**

75 per cent of people who go on a weight-reducing diet give up without losing very much, and of the remaining 25 per cent, or less, few manage to maintain their weight-reduction for very long.

Although it is tempting, therefore, to conclude that diets don't work, a more accurate assessment is that most people lack the sufficient will-power needed to make them work. Contrary to popular belief, as well as to the sales hype that surrounds the publication of each new diet book, there is no wonder diet which surpasses all others in its ability to help you slim. All diets work fundamentally by restricting Calorie (kilojoule) intake, and the more limited this intake, the more rapid the rate of weight-loss.

**Why diets fail**

The choice of modern slimming diets is vast, the various permutations of foods you may or may not eat as a means of restricting Calories (kilojoules) varies greatly. However, since individual requirements differ widely, there is no single diet that will work for everybody. Successful slimming is ultimately dependent on finding a diet which will suit you – your tastes, your goals, your lifestyle, your temperament and body type. The review of today's popular diets included in this chapter should help give you some idea of the different types which can help you lose weight according to your individual needs.

While anyone can lose weight on a diet, few manage to maintain their new low weight. Strictly speaking, in the long run the majority of diets fail because excess weight-loss through dieting is inevitably regained either partially or completely. This is particularly true for anyone who has lost a lot of weight very quickly, through following a very restricted or gimmicky 'crash' diet. Hunger, boredom, loss of will-power, frustration or disappointment at not being able to lose weight fast enough or reach one's target weight, are the most common reasons given by slimmers for giving up their diet.

The promise of rapid weight-loss accounts for the immense popularity of many modern low-Calorie (kilojoule) diets. Their appeal, however, tends to be largely short-lived for one very simple reason: those excess pounds (kilos) will only disappear rapidly at the very beginning of a restrictive diet. At this stage it is not fat, but excess water, bound up with glycogen (carbohydrate stores) and protein, drawn from the tissues as an energy source, that is being eliminated by the body. The diets may initially lose five or six pounds (2 kg), or even more in fluid. He or she then reaches a frustrating but inevitable stage where the rate of weight-reduction slows down considerably and usually settles at around one or two pounds (450 g–1 kg) per week. Gloom may supersede euphoria. It is during this difficult phase that all the will-power and perseverance in the world are needed, with the ultimate goal weight and new slimline body firmly fixed in the mind. But the rewards, for those who do persevere, usually more than make up for the slog and self-denial.

## Changing bad habits permanently

In order to attain a permanent lower weight, especially if you are more than nine pounds (4 kg) to a stone (14 lbs/6 kg) overweight, a sensible, balanced modification of everyday eating habits will ultimately pay greater dividends than adopting unhealthy crash diets, skipping meals or starving yourself. Permanent weight-reduction can only result from changing bad eating habits for good ones. This means, for instance, cutting down or eliminating sweets or candy, chocolate, sugary snacks, fried foods etc., and substituting for them non-fattening wholefoods, fruit and vegetables, thereby re-educating one's attitudes to food generally. Someone who manages to adopt healthy eating patterns as an integral and permanent part of their life, stands a far greater chance of successfully losing surplus weight – and keeping it off for good.

Slow weight-loss, at the rate of say one–two pounds (450 g–1 kg) per week, is less likely to be regained when you begin to eat normally than weight which is lost too quickly. If you have managed to lose a lot of weight over a short period as a result of following a very restricted diet, then it follows that when you resume anything resembling a normal pattern of eating some, if not all of that weight will be regained. This explains the sense of following, as far as possible, a healthy *balanced* diet that nonetheless eliminates obviously fattening foods and beverages.

Most women will lose weight on 1,000 Calories (4,200 kilojoules) a day, most men, on 1,500 Calories (6,300 kilojoules) a day, because the body needs more energy than this to function normally. Cutting out approximately 500 Calories (2,100 kilojoules) a day from your diet should lead to the loss of about one pound (450 g) per week. It is worth remembering, too, that by increasing your Calorie (kilojoule)output through exercise you may also lose weight more quickly without having to resort to extremes of dietary deprivation.

## THE ELUSIVE 'X' FACTOR

Successful dieting depends as much on will-power, determination and calorie-reduction as on that mysterious 'x factor' individual metabolism. This is the major imponderable that continues to puzzle scientists as much as it infuriates fat people and slimmers, their lives made miserable by the inability to attain a lower goal weight, in spite of stringent dieting. Why it is that some people gain or regain weight easily, while others lose weight or remain slim even though they eat large quantities of food, remains a conundrum yet to be resolved. Are we really what we eat? The old adage that people get fat just because they eat more seems overly simplistic in the light of recent studies of dieting and weight-loss. These studies have produced findings which go some way to explain the idiosyncracies of individual and fluctuating body-weight.

**Brown fat**

The discovery of the phenomenon of brown adipose tissue lends credence to the rather depressing theory that we are all congenitally predisposed to be either fat or thin. Tests carried out on rats show that brown adipose tissue located at specific sites of the body, e.g. between the shoulder blades and around the vital organs, contains a high concentration of highly metabolically active fat cells. These act as the body's 'furnace', burning up Calories (kilojoules) rapidly to provide energy and body heat. Brown fat is distinguished by an increased flow of blood through it, and the extra large and efficient nuclei of the cell, the mitochondria, which contain brown pigments and are responsible for fully converting food into energy.

The amount of brown fat in humans and animals is proportionately far lower than ordinary fat – white fat makes up about 22 per cent of body weight, brown fat only about one per cent or less – but research suggests that in certain individuals brown fat may be metabolically ineffective, or present in smaller quantities. This discovery certainly helps to explain why people seem to fall into 'naturally' slim or plump categories. Research is currently under way to discover whether stores of brown fat, which is also thought to become less efficient in later life, can be made to function more efficiently with the use of thermogenic drugs.

The search is now on for a drug that could act only on brown fat cells, perhaps via the central nervous system, without harmful side-effects. Stress chemicals such as noradrenaline, and nicotine in tobacco and caffeine in coffee, are known to have a stimulating effect on brown fat. Meanwhile, studies carried out in America indicate that rats fed on a high-fat meal produce less heat and burn up fewer calories than those fed a high-carbohydrate meal. This difference is in part attributable to the metabolic activity of brown fat. Calorie for Calorie (kilojoule for kilojoule), therefore, high-fat foods are considered likely to cause greater weight-gain than high-carbohydrate foods.

## The set point theory

Many dieters are familiar with the plateau stage of weight-loss, whereby after losing a significant amount of weight over a few weeks the weight then simply sticks, in spite of stringent dietary restrictions. The inability to shed those extra stubborn pounds prevents many slimmers from attaining their ideal goal weight. Another contributory factor in diet 'failures' is also persistent hunger. Both phenomena have been attributed to the theory that we are all born with an inbuilt metabolic rate, or set point, at which our bodies function at optimum level. Implicit in this proposition is the fact that we are genetically programmed to carry a certain quantity of fat and our bodies will resists the effect of dieting in an effort to maintain this quota.

As weight is lost, signals sent out by the brain (principally the hypothalamus) increase feelings of hunger and the metabolic rate slows down in order to conserve Calories (kilojoules). Dieting can lower the body's basic metabolic rate and studies at Queen Elizabeth College in London show that long-term dieters become metabolically adapted to eating less food, with the result that the rate of weight reduction then decreases. There is no mystery about this, since a body that weighs less obviously requires less energy than one that weighs more.

Some researchers suggest a rather neat corollary to this adaptation syndrome, namely that abandoning the diet results in rapid 'rebound' weight-gain. The reason for this is either that the metabolic rate is too sluggish to burn up extra Calories (kilojoules) or, as some studies suggest, the body has to struggle to regain its former weight and establish a normal metabolic rate. Trying to maintain a reduced body-weight by taking in fewer Calories (kilojoules) than normal seems to place the metabolism under stress, the argument goes, and rebound 'binge' eating after dieting reflects a response to that stress.

**Easy does it, the best method**
What all this suggests, though based as yet on empirical rather than hard scientific evidence, is that opting for very rapid weight-reduction by going on a crash diet may cause the metabolic rate to become more unstable than it would as a result of losing weight slowly and steadily at a rate of about one to two pounds (450 g–1 kg) a week. Easing oneself slowly and gently into a different, but balanced, eating pattern may prove less of a shock to the metabolic rate and the brain's appetite centre. Ultimately, this enables you to maintain the new lower weight more easily.

Proponents of the theory that dieting can make you more liable to put on weight, also argue that weight-loss can be achieved more effectively through upping energy output, i.e., by increasing exercise. There is some evidence to suggest that taking fairly vigorous and regular exercise can raise metabolism significantly over short periods and help you burn off more Calories (kilojoules). However, whether increasing physical activity can permanently alter the body's metabolic rate, remains as yet unproven. What does seem certain is that our metabolic rate is determined genetically. Scientists hope one day to develop a drug which could be used to crank up a defective or sluggish metabolism without harmful side-effects.

Exactly how the body regulates itself to compensate for fluctuating weight-loss is a mystery yet to be unravelled. Scientists believe fat cells play a key role in signalling the brain to switch hunger signals up or down, according to the level of fat they contain. Fat cells do not alter in numbers, but they do swell or shrink according to weight lost or gained, probably releasing chemical 'messengers' into the bloodstream which directly influence the brain.

### Alpha and Beta receptors

Achieving one's goal weight is not necessarily the same thing as acquiring an ideal figure. Surplus fat often tends to accumulate more noticeably on hips, bottoms and thighs, clinging on stubbornly long after excess flesh has dropped away elsewhere. Losing weight, but not inches (centimetres), is often the bane of dieting. This is especially true for women, who are often unable to reduce surplus fat below the waist, compared to men who achieve a more uniform weight-loss.

Scientists believe the key to the problem lies in the types of fat cells we carry, in particular their inbuilt 'codes' which determine how easily they release or retain fat. Fat cells carry two different types of receptors on their surface: Alpha 2 Receptors inhibit the breakdown of fat, Beta 1 Receptors stimulate its release. The ratio between these two different varieties is somewhat uneven in women, who carry more fat-retaining Alpha 2 cells in areas below the waist than men. For men, this type of fat is concentrated mainly around the stomach, accounting for the familiar 'pot belly'.

Like brown fat and preset metabolism, the type of fat cells we carry are almost certainly inherited and there is little you can do to fundamentally alter your particular quota and location of stubborn fat. Work is currently taking place to perfect a drug which could be used to either block Alpha Receptors, or stimulate Beta Receptors into releasing more fat, but realisation of such substances for general use is certainly a long way off. Until then, some experts believe that, once again, taking regular exercise may help to encourage a more efficient breakdown of fat.

—— A REVIEW OF TODAY'S MOST POPULAR DIETS ——

*Note*

If you have any past or present health problems, you must check with your doctor before beginning any slimming diet. The more this diet deviates from your normal eating habits, the more important it is to follow this rule.

**The Atkins Diet**

A high protein/high fat, minimal carbohydrate diet that dispenses with calorie counting. Instead, dieters are supposed to test their urine using paper dip-sticks to assess the level of ketosis, a chemical indication of how effectively the body is burning up fat.

This diet, which is high in saturated fats and cholesterol, very low in carbohydrate, basically contravenes all today's medical recommendations for a healthy, well-balanced and moderate diet. A diet which relies almost exclusively on a plethora of fat seems an anomaly at a time when doctors are attempting to make us more conscious of the rising rate of heart disease. It is, after all, hard to ignore increasing medical research which lays the blame for arteriosclerosis and coronary disease, as well as some forms of cancer, fairly and squarely on a diet high in rich fatty food.

The fact that the Atkins Diet does make you lose weight rapidly – initially at the rate of about ten pounds (4.5 kg) in one week – and without deprivation, cannot be denied. Weight-loss is based on the premise that, if you restrict your carbohydrate intake to almost zero, your body will use up fat for energy rather than storing it, and at the same time also tap accumulated body fat for extra fuel.

According to Dr Atkins, the proof of this 'internal combustion' lies in the amount of ketones excreted in the urine. Ketones are like ash, the unburnt chemicals left behind when fats are burnt. Their presence in the urine shows that the body is metabolising its own store of fat. Dieters are advised to check their urine daily to make sure they are still producing chemicals. The test is carried out using special paper tester strips which turn purple if your body is in ketosis.

While ketones do curb your appetite and so help you lose weight, over longer periods they can prove harmful, creating acidity, irritating the kidneys and allowing your blood sugar level to plummet. For this reason the Atkins diet consists of just one week of 'zero carbohydrate' menus, naturally easing off to admit more carbohydrate foods such as fruit and vegetables, during which time you must continuously test your urine for ketones.

Cutting out carbohydrates, says Dr Atkins, also triggers the secretion of a chemical called Fat Mobilising Hormone (FMH) which stokes up the body's fat-burning mechanism even further. Overweight people, he maintains, have a deficiency of FMH because they are fundamentally 'allergic' to carbohydrates, storing them away as fat instead of using them up as energy. It is a spurious claim if you bear in mind that many people *do* manage to lose weight on a high carbohydrate, low fat diet. Just as significant is the fact that the American Medical Association states that there is as yet no scientific evidence to prove that FMH exists, or is produced when you starve yourself of carbohydrates.

Altogether Dr Atkins uses some pretty specious arguments to bolster his high fat slimming theory. While he rightly condemns sugar, sweet food and alcohol for causing ill health and obesity, he chooses to overlook the dangers to the heart and arteries of eating a lot of saturated fats and cholesterol. He also tells dieters to beware of the 'hidden' sugar and carbohydrate content in such important staple foods as fruit and fruit juices. The very fact that Dr Atkins prescribes very large vitamin supplements to patients embarking on the diet, surely indicates its degree of nutritional imbalance.

However, on the positive side, provided you are not pregnant, do not suffer from kidney problems and have no history of thrombosis, heart or circulatory trouble, you may find the Atkins diet one of the cushiest ways of losing weight. Ultimately, however, it does nothing to help dieters towards healthy eating patterns, or to re-educate their tastebuds to appreciate 'cleaner' foods. It is, therefore, very rapidly losing ground to the healthy, more streamlined, high protein diets like the Scarsdale, or high fibre diets like the F Plan.

### Verdict
*Weight loss potential:*
Excellent – fast and noticeable for the first week or two.
*Deprivation factor:*
Very low. Boredom and hunger pangs are unlikely to be a problem, provided you like rich food.
*Interest value:*
Also considerable, especially if you enjoy rich foods such as dairy produce.
*Recommended for:*
Only those in good health with no history of arteriosclerosis, thrombosis, high cholesterol and triglyceride (fat) levels. The diet is excellent and non-punitive for people who socialise and eat out a lot.
*Nutritional aspect*
* Ketosis occurs when most of the body's energy is being derived from fat but it's not a reliable measure of the efficacy of

a weight reducing diet.

* The assumption that a low carbohydrate/high fat intake stimulates removal of body fat is not based on scientific fact.

* Although high in fat, this diet probably still results in the user eating fewer calories than usual and this is likely to be the reason for weight-loss rather than ketosis.

* Use of dipsticks adds novelty value but is not an accurate indication of metabolic processes.

* Mild ketosis is unlikely to be harmful to a healthy individual but recommending high intakes of fat flies in the face of current guidelines for healthy eating.

This diet is unlikely to change basic eating habits and will almost inevitably cause constipation.

*Dietary details:*

The Atkins diet consists of five weekly stages:

1) Days 1–7, no carbohydrate intake (i.e. bread, potatoes, crispbread), only very low Calorie (kilojoule) rolls are permitted. Permitted foods include all meats, fish, poultry, eggs, cheese, mixed salad, clear soups, zero-Calorie (kilojoule) drinks. Ketostick test after five days should show a high rate of ketosis, i.e. the stick will turn purple.

2) At this stage you add a little carbohydrate to the diet, no more than ¾ oz (15–20 g). Suggested sources: vegetables, cottage cheese or ricotta, nuts, seeds, seafood, organ meats, sausage.

3) More carbohydrate can be added to the diet, preferably in the form of vegetables, and perhaps the occassional alcoholic drink. If the ketostick does not turn purple however, you must return to stage 1. In this way you learn to assess your own 'critical carbohydrate level' when the stick no longer turns purple. The idea is to eat just enough carbohydrate to allow ketosis to continue.

4) Fruit may now be added to the diet and half a slice of bread. At this stage the ketostick should show at least a mauvy tinge.

Modify carbohydrate intake accordingly.

5) The final maintenance stage, where Atkins advises 'bending of the diet without breaking it'. Previously forbidden foods can be added, without ketostick testing, till weight-loss slows down to one pound a week or less. At this point, to maintain your ideal weight you should choose which carbohydrate foods you crave most (with the exception of all sweets and sugars, which should be banned completely), and eat them in moderation.

## The Scarsdale medical diet

This is a high protein, low carbohydrate and fat diet. It encourages weight-loss on the basis that, unlike fat and carbohydrate, which are stored as fat, protein is used up as metabolic fuel, inducing ketosis (see Atkins diet). The diet consists of two separate stages: an initial, very rigid and fixed regimen aimed at promoting a two-week rapid weight-loss, followed by a two-week Keep Trim programme, when weight-loss is minimal or stops altogether.

The logic of this diet is supported by a rather tenuous theory that, since a protein molecule is large and chemically complex, the body has to use up extra energy to digest it. This means that you may burn about 275 Calories (1,155 kilojoules) more per day then on a diet of the same Calorie (kilojoule) intake taken from fats and carbohydrates.

The so-called 'dynamics' of protein mean that if you stick to meat, fish, eggs, low fat cheese and salad, you should rapidly burn up and 'melt away' excess body fat. To a certain extent, of course, this is exactly how a high protein diet works, which accounts for its instant appeal. If, as on the Scarsdale Diet, you are not eating enough carbohydrates and fat to supply your body with sufficient calories, then your system first draws on stored body tissue to act as fuel. It is little wonder, therefore, that you can lose an average of one pound (450 g) a day, or 20 to 40 pounds (9–18 kg) a fortnight.

But if this seems impressive, remember that this instant and rapid loss is due, very largely, to the reduction of the water content inside and outside the body's cells. This is an essential part of the body's adaptation process in response to restricted Calorie (kilojoule) intake. It is as well to bear in mind that when weight is lost rapidly, it is not fat stores which are being used up as a primary source of energy but rather glycogen and lean tissue, including muscle.

Compared to many earlier, low carbohydrate diets, the Scarsdale is relatively well-balanced, allowing you to eat fruit, vegetables, small quantities of low-Calorie (kilojoule) bread and dairy produce. However, lack of carbohydrate may frequently be the cause of tiredness, dizziness, irritability and similar conditions generally associated with low blood sugar levels. It does not contain enough carbohydrate to make it a safe and feasible eating plan for more than a fortnight.

The rigid 'if it's Tuesday, it must be fish' format is one of the main, if monotonous, features of the Scarsdale Diet. Perversely, this is what makes the diet work for the majority of people who try it. There is no room for mealtime manoeuvring, and you are supposed to follow daily menus down to the last lettuce leaf. By making up your mind for you, the agony and indecision is taken out of planning meals. However, more ambiguous is exactly how much you should eat at every meal. One of the attractions, as well as the drawbacks, of the Scarsdale diet is its avoidance of Calorie (kilojoule)-counting, with the apparent licence to over-eat. After all, 'plenty of lean meat' has different interpretations for different people, no matter how often the instructions tell you not to gorge yourself. It is also a fact that any surplus protein that your body doesn't use up as energy is stored as fat.

However, there is little doubt that the Scarsdale is one of the most pleasant and uncomplicated two-week diets to follow if you want to lose weight quickly without suffering hunger pangs or becoming unsociable. Maintaining that loss is another matter, since the moment you adjust the diet to include a wider range of foods you will incur a greater appetite, stop losing fluid and begin storing fat once again.

The diet works best for people following an alternate two weeks strict regime, two weeks trim routine for about eight weeks. Once you have reached your desired weight you will have to follow the keep trim programme for evermore. Keeping weight off is far more difficult than losing it on this programme, so it is really only effective during the strict two-week phase, which could prove dangerous if you remain on it for longer. An ideal diet, therefore, for anyone about eight to ten pounds (3–5 kg) overweight.

**Verdict**
*Weight-loss potential:*
Excellent – fast and noticeable initially, although this is largely due to water-loss. After initial weight-reduction, the rate slows down considerably.
*Deprivation factor:*
Hunger pangs are minimal, and since you do not have to count Calories (kilojoules) you should be able to eat enough at each meal to satisfy your appetite.
*Interest value:*
Adhering to the initial two-week reducing regime can be boring, but you can swap the different food schedules, i.e. eat lunch-time food at dinner and vice versa. *The Scarsdale Book* does include a wide variety of different types of menus which provide an opportunity to broaden the diet after the two-week, strict reduction programme.
*Recommended for:*
Anyone who dislikes counting Calories (kilojoules), gets hungry on a diet, eats out a lot, and enjoys meat, fish and other

high protein foods and does not crave sweet, starchy foods. It will also suit those prepared to pay extra money for lean meat etc, and whose lifestyle allows them to eat the precise combination of foods stipulated in the diet.

*Nutritional aspect:*

This high protein/low fat diet works because it's basically low in Calories (kilojoules). Popular claims that high protein diets can work metabolic magic are largely unproven. This diet is low in fat which makes it a healthier alternative to the Atkins diet but its fibre content is undesirably low and again likely to cause constipation. Initial high weight-losses are due mostly to the loss of body water and lean tissue rather than fat and likely to be regained rapidly once the diet has been abandoned.

*One typical week on the Scarsdale Diet:*

*Breakfast every day* – Half a grapefruit – if not available, use fruit in season. One slice of high protein bread, toasted, no spread added, coffee/tea (no sugar, cream or milk).

*Monday, Lunch* – Assorted cold cuts (your choice, lean meats, chicken, turkey, tongue, lean beef etc.) tomatoes sliced, grilled or stewed, coffee/tea/diet soda.

*Dinner* – Fish or shellfish of any kind, combination salad, as many green vegetables as you wish. One slice of high protein bread, toasted. Grapefruit – if not available, fruits in season. Coffee/tea.

*Tuesday, Lunch* – Fruit salad, any combination of fruits, as much as you want. Coffee/tea.

*Dinner* – Plenty of grilled lean hamburger, salad of tomatoes, lettuce, celery, olives or cucumber. Coffee/tea.

*Wednesday, Lunch* – Tuna fish or salmon salad (oil drained off) with lemon and vinegar dressing. Grapefruit or melon or fruit in season. Coffee/tea.

*Dinner* – Sliced roast lamb without fat, salad of lettuce, tomatoes, cucumber, celery. Coffee/tea.

*Thursday, Lunch* – Two eggs, any style but not fried (no fat to be used in cooking), low fat cottage cheese or ricotta, courgettes (zucchini) or string beans or sliced or stewed tomatoes. One slice of high protein bread toasted. Coffee/tea.

*Dinner* – Roast, grilled (broiled) or barbecued chicken – as much as you want, with skin and visible fat removed. Plenty of spinach, green peppers, string beans. Coffee/tea.

*Friday, Lunch* – Assorted cheese slices, spinach, all you want. One slice of high protein bread, toasted. Coffee/tea.

*Dinner* – Fish or shellfish, combination salad and as many fresh vegetables as you wish, including cold, diced, cooked vegetables. One slice of high protein bread, toasted. Coffee/tea.

*Saturday, Lunch* – Fruit salad, as much as you want. Coffee/tea.

*Dinner* – Roast turkey or chicken, salad of tomato and lettuce, grapefruit or fruit in season. Coffee/tea.

*Sunday, Lunch* – Cold or hot turkey or chicken, tomatoes, carrots, cooked cabbage, broccoli or cauliflower, grapefruit or fruit in season. Coffee/tea.

*Dinner* – Plenty of grilled steak, without any fat. Salad of lettuce, cucumber, celery, tomato sliced or cooked. Coffee/tea.

### The Pritikin diet

A high complex (i.e. unrefined) carbohydrate, low protein, very low fat diet which includes a high percentage of vegetable fibre. Geared as much to disease-prevention as weight-loss, the diet was devised as part of a treatment package including exercise for cardiac patients at the Longevity Research Institute in California. The late Nathan Pritikin was a medical maverick who firmly believed we must learn to cut out all but the smallest amounts of fat, protein and sugar from our diet. This leaves fibre-rich complex carbohydrates – and the diet is a staggering 80 per cent carbohydrate, 10 per cent fat, 10 per cent protein.

An increasing number of medical experts are beginning to concur with Pritikin, and theoretically the diet is perfectly in tune with the health-conscious trend toward vegetarianism, reduced consumption of meat and dairy produce, and increased fibre intake. Ten years ago, the punishingly low fat and protein levels and high percentage of bulky carbohydrates wouldn't have done much to inspire the taste buds of anyone still hooked on vast quantities of meat as part of their everyday diet.

Yet as more and more of us shun red meat, fat and sugar, and explore a wider variety of vegetarian recipes, the Pritikin Diet might not appear so unattractive. In reality it is thoroughly a killjoy.

Apart from cutting out some staple protein foods like milk, eggs and cheese, as well as polyunsaturated oils and margarines and reducing salt drastically, it firmly eliminates coffee, tea and practically all alcohol. What's more, your limited weekly allowance of fish or meat amounts to a meagre 24 ounces (600 g). So it is a spartan regime, to say the least.

By avoiding nearly all forms of fat and animal protein and substituting instead raw and cooked vegetables, pulses, roots, grains and fruit, Nathan Pritikin claims that, provided we begin early enough in life, we can avoid most common diseases. Heart failure, due to clogging up of the arteries with rich, fatty food, is obviously one of the targeted diseases. If you are a strict vegetarian you have a head start, since Pritikin believes in using fish and meat only as accompaniment to your main vegetable dish, rather than the other way round. At best, however, it is an indigestible, inflexible regime – no matter how you try to embellish and combine its basic ingredients.

If you are a nibbler it is a great diet, as you are required to eat four pounds (2 kg) of food a day in eight meals. But this is a lot when you consider that many dieters eat roughly four pounds (2 kg) of food *a week*. From this quantity you only take in 600 to 700 Calories (2,520–2,940 kilojoules), as most of the food consists of vegetables. On this spartan programme overweight patients at the Longevity Centre apparently lose an average of 34 pounds (15 kg) in just under four weeks.

Probably the most positive aspect of the Pritikin diet is that it makes you look at fruit and vegetables in a different light. Apart from becoming more aware of different varieties and interesting ways in which to cook them, it also teaches you to eat small amounts at frequent intervals. In this way, you overcome the habit of 'pigging out' on one blockbusting meal, once a day.

Menus are planned to provide either 600, 850, 1,000 or 1,200 Calories (2,520, 3,570, 4,200 or 5,040 kilojoules) each day for two weeks, depending on your needs. Although many of the recipes included are tasty and interestingly varied, the overall impression is one of blandness for anyone who enjoys meat, dairy produce and sweet foods.

## Verdict

*Weight-loss potential:*
Excellent, especially on the 600 Calorie (2,520 kilojoule), maximum weight-loss diet, which leads to a rapid initial reduction of three or four pounds (1–2 kg) a week, due to loss of water. The usual amount of weight lost by overweight people at the Pritikin Centre is just under a stone (14 lbs/6 kg) in one month.

*Deprivation factor:*
Minimal, unless you regard tea, coffee and the occasional glass of wine as less a luxury than a necessity to civilised living, or if you crave rich, fatty foods, meat, fish and sweets or candy. However, you are allowed to nibble as frequently as necessary, provided you stick to raw vegetable snacks. Hunger should not be a problem because of the emphasis on unrefined wholefoods such as beans, bread, potatoes, pasta. These all fill you up rapidly and for extended periods.

*Interest value:*
Tremendous, if you don't regard meat or dairy produce as

integral to a full and varied diet.

*Recommended for:*

Anyone who is health-conscious, a vegetarian or non-meat eater who enjoys eating raw vegetables, salads, pulses, seeds, wholemeal foods.

*Nuritional aspect:*

The high fibre, low fat content of the Pritikin diet adds up to a healthy way of eating providing you can cope with the bulk and possible monotony. It's difficult to eat too many Calories (kilojoules) on this diet and it should ensure an adequate intake of protein, vitamins and minerals. Healthy as it is, the Pritikin diet is probably too restrictive for most people to follow on a long term basis.

*Sample menu from the Pritikin Diet:*

*Breakfast* – Half a grapefruit, bowl of cooked wholegrain cereal with fruit, skimmed milk and bran.

*Lunch* – Bowl of vegetable soup. Large wholemeal bread sandwich containing green salad, pickled vegetables, sprinkled with vinegar, lemon and bran.

*Dinner* – Meat soup, steamed broccoli, courgettes (zucchini), brown rice, salad, wholemeal bread, stewed apples, yoghurt.

*Snacks* – Three snacks of either fruit, salad or wholemeal sandwiches.

*Foods not permitted on the Pritikin Diet:*

Fats

Oils

Sugars

Fat Meat

Offal

Milk (except skimmed milk)

Egg yolks

Cheeses (except less than one per cent fat by weight)

Nuts (except chestnuts)

Seeds (except grains)

Soya beans
Avocados
Olives
Cooked, tinned, or frozen food with sugar
Jam (Jelly)
Syrup
Grain products made with added fats or egg yolks, including some pastas
Salt in excess of 0.2 oz (4 g) per day
Mayonnaise
Sandwich spreads
Gravies
Sauces
Most dessert items (containing fats, oils, sugars, egg yolks)
Sweets, chocolate, candy
Alcoholic drinks (an occasional glass of light white wine is allowed)
Tea, coffee, cola drinks

**The F-Plan diet**
This high-fibre, low-Calorie diet requires both Calorie (kilo-joule) and fibre-counting. You are advised to eat between 1,000 and 1,500 Calories (4,200 and 6,300 kilojoules) and between 1½–1¾ oz (35 and 50 g) of fibre a day, which is twice most people's normal consumption.

There is, of course, nothing dramatically new about this type of eating programme, which is very similar to the Pritikin diet. Neither is there anything original about its findings, based as they are on a considerable amount of nutritional and medical research carried out by such pioneers as Dr Denis Burkitt, Dr Hugh Trowell, Dr Alick Walker and Surgeon Captain Sir Hugh Cleave. These doctors worked extensively in different rural areas of southern Africa, and all have produced very persuasive evidence for the protective health benefits of dietary fibre. There seems little doubt that there is a strong correlation between the high incidence of western degenerative diseases, including obesity, and a diet high in saturated fats and refined foods. Recent medical recommendations all emphasise the need to cut down on these while increasing our intake of fibre-rich wholefoods, vegetables and fruit. The F-Plan diet is therefore based on sound, sensible rules of healthy eating.

According to Audrey Eyton, originator of the diet, eating extra fibre will help you lose weight in two ways. Firstly, fibre-rich foods are bulky and filling, so a little goes a long way and you tend to eat less, while avoiding hunger pangs for longer periods. Secondly, perhaps the more contentious claim is that, since fibre represents that part of plants which is not digested, fibre-rich foods pass through the intestines more rapidly, allowing a certain amount of Calories (kilojoules) to be excreted in the stool (faeces). Just what percentage of one's intake of Calories (kilojoules) on a high-fibre diet might be eliminated in this way is however unclear, although Audrey Eyton states that 'tests indicate that the increased Calorie (kilojoule) content of the faeces amounts to nearly 10 per cent when people follow high-fibre diets'.

That these foods are filling and stem appetite, however, cannot be denied, which accounts for the popularity of the diet. In spite of the undoubted healthgiving benefits of wholefoods, some doctors have recently expressed concern that eating too much fibre can lead to certain mineral and vitamin deficiencies.

**Verdict**

*The weight-loss potential:*
Moderate to good. The diet encourages steady reduction of about one to three pounds (450 g to 1.3 kg) a week in weight, nothing more dramatic. Maintaining weight-loss is easier on

this diet than on other high-protein diets.

*Deprivation factor:*

Very low. The diet is not killjoy or doctrinaire. Hunger pangs between meals and lack of satisfaction after meals are rare, because food provides bulk and fills you up for long periods, maintaining a steady balance of blood sugar. Tea and coffee are allowed and ½ pint (300 ml) of milk must be consumed on the diet. A little alcohol is also allowed.

*Interest value:*

High. The meal plans are well-balanced and flexible, and recipes are varied and interesting, including meat and fish, ideas for sandwiches, non-fattening desserts, quick snacks and meals on toast. Anyone who has dismissed the F-Plan as consisting only of endless variations on a theme of beans and bran, will get a pleasant surprise.

*Recommended for:*

Anyone who wants a painless, non-masochistic but effective route to weight-lose. More than most other popular slimming diets, this one is likely to help dieters not only lose weight but simultaneously re-educate their eating habits for longer periods by encouraging a healthy, relatively well-balanced diet.

*Nutritional aspect:*

A basically sound and sensible way to reduce weight that fits in with today's ideas about healthy eating. Although excessive intakes of fibre can reduce the absorption of certain minerals it's unlikely to happen with this diet providing a good variety of foods are eaten.

Weight-loss will probably be less dramatic, compared with other diets, but is more easily maintained.

**The Beverly Hills diet**

This high carbohydrate, low protein diet supposedly encourages eating and abolishes hunger. It involves eating according to strict rules: proteins are only eaten with other proteins and fats, carbohydrates with other carbohydrates and fats with fats or carbohydrates, while fruit must be eaten on its own. Fruit forms the basis of this diet during the first ten days. Judy Mazel, who formulated the regime, claims that the enzymes in tropical fruits such as papaya and pineapple burn up fat and digest superfluous protein which is clogging up the system.

Most of the claims made by the author have been dismissed by doctors and nutritionists as misleading, as they have little scientific basis. It has not been proven, for example, that fats or protein block the digestion of other nutrients, or that enzymes in food speed up the elimination of other foods. Fruit is seen as the salvation of anyone who likes to binge on fattening food and every food binge must be followed, says Mazel, by eating nothing but fruit again for the next three days.

What this diet represents, therefore, is simply another variation on alternate binge/deprivation eating, contrary to all accepted rules of healthy eating. It therefore does nothing to re-educate eating patterns and help the dieter develop a taste for healthier, nutritious, less fattening foods.

The claim that fat represents no more than 'undigested food' is totally fallacious. *All* food before it can be used as fuel or laid down as fat first undergoes fundamental digestive processes. If, as Judy Mazel says, one of the most obvious symptoms of indigestion is fat, why should so many thin people suffer indigestion while many fat ones don't? Mazel even implies that artifical sweeteners are fattening because 'these are based on chemicals the body cannot digest'. Since, except in extremely rare cases, the body automatically produces its own digestive enzymes which break down various foods into their constituent parts as part of the digestive process, it is unlikely that the extra enzymes ingested from tropical fruit are likely to do the job faster or more efficiently.

However, the diet scores in offering a delicious fruit-only diet, on the lines of an upmarket nature cure regime. This certainly leads to considerable weight-loss, even though much of it is due to fluid reduction.

The reason for the 'best seller' status of this particular diet is undoubtedly the inbuilt licence to resume eating exactly what you want again after the first punitive fortnight.

### Verdict
*Weight-loss potential:*
Good in the first ten to 14 days; as much as one pound (450 g) a day will be lost initially.
*Deprivation factor:*
Considerable over the first fruit-only period. Thereafter, you can alternately gorge and then deprive yourself, by veering between two extremes of eating.
*Interest value:*
Excellent, provided you like sweet, exotic fruits such as papaya, mango, pineapple and can afford to buy them, if, of course, you are lucky enough to be able to find them in the first place throughout the year.
*Recommended for:*
Anyone who likes fruit and is prepared to hunt and pay high prices for it, especially out of season. Not for diabetics, people with blood sugar problems, pregnant women.
*Nutritional aspect:*
A con! There's no evidence to back up the claim that enzymes in certain foods help to break down or burn up body fat stores. Weight-loss on this diet is the result of a low Calorie (kilojoule) intake. Deficiencies are likely to result with prolonged use and the laxative effects of excessively high fruit intakes could be an unpleasant side-effect.

## The Rotation diet

A rapid weight-loss diet based on alternating your Calorie (kilojoule) intake over a three week period. For the first three days you consume 600 Calories (2,520 kilojoules), stepping this up to 900 Calories (3,780 kilojoules) for the next four days, then sticking to 1200 Calories (5,040 kilojoules) for the following week. Finally, during the third week you switch again to the 600/900 Calorie (2,520/3,780 kilojoule) rotation.

Men follow an alternative 1200/1500/1800 Calorie (5,040/6,300/7,560 kilojoule) rotation. According to its innovator, Dr Martin Katahn, women following this form of synchronised stop-go Calorie (kilojoule) controlled eating lose on average two-thirds to one pound (300 to 450 g) per day over 21 days while men may lose more. The diet is well balanced, low in saturated fats, high in fibre-rich carbohydrates, lean meat, fish, poultry, fruit and vegetables. The diet has been devised very sensibly taking into account two depressing and universal problems that afflict the majority of dieters – insufficient initial weight-loss and, in the case of those who do lose a lot of weight on a 'crash diet', the tendency to put it all back again when near normal eating habits are resumed after the diet. Both these problems are often a direct result of the body's tendency to lower its base metabolic rate in response to a prolonged (i.e. 2–3 weeks) period of drastically reduced food intake. This metabolic adaptation, an inbuilt evolutionary mechanism probably developed by man to survive periods of famine works against modern day slimmers by slowing down the rate at which large amounts of weight can be lost. Following the premise that a very restricted Calorie (kilojoule) intake is essential for rapid weight reduction, the diet ingeniously aims to secure those losses initially while preventing the body from becoming accustomed to longterm, undeviating low Calorie (kilojoule) input, so decreasing its metabolic rate. By alternately raising and lowering the amount of Calories (kilojoules) eaten, the idea is, on the contrary, to raise the metabolic rate, ideally increasing a person's ability to eat normally after the diet without regaining weight. Dr Katahn claims that once they have lost weight most people eating a judicious choice of healthy foods and taking plenty of exercise should eat 20 per cent more Calories (kilojoules) per day than they do normally and not gain weight. Wishful thinking this may be, especially for those whose 'normal' diet includes cakes, fried potatoes and chocolate bars, but in fact this is a neatly logical hypothesis which fits in well with current 'setpoint' and 'dieting makes you fat' theories. Regular daily exercise is strongly recommended as an adjunct as this helps further in raising metabolism. Another point in favour of this chop-change system of dieting is that it obviates much of the boredom, and sense of deprivation inherent in many rapid weight-loss diets and therefore does a lot to boost motivation to stick to it.

After a break of a week or a month, anyone with more weight to lose may resume the diet. Losses of over 70 pounds (34 kg) are recorded on the Rotation diet. Diabetics however must not follow the 600/900 Calorie (2,520/3,780 kilojoule) eating plans and are advised to follow higher Calorie (kilojoule) permutations. With the F-Plan, this ranks as probably the most interesting, effective and nutritionally sound weight-loss scheme around, and will suit those people who find their weight 'sticks' at about 5 or 10 lbs (2.25–4.5 kg) above their desired weight.

### Verdict
*Weight-loss potential:*
Excellent. 5 lbs (2.25 kg) or more during the first and third week, about 2½ lbs (1 kg) over the second middle week, with higher rates for men. You can hope to lose an average of 12½ lbs (5 kg) over 21 days. Regular exercise is recommended to accelerate weight loss and prevent weight gain.

*Deprivation factor:*
Because Calorie (kilojoule) restriction is sporadic not continuous, this is far less punitive than other rapid weight-loss
regimes. Hunger may be a problem mostly during the 600
Calorie (2,520 kilojoule) days, obviously least of all during 1200
Calorie (5,040 kilojoule) days. As with the Pritikin diet, there is
a comprehensive range of low Calorie (kilojoule) fruits and
raw vegetables which you are permitted to eat as snacks
throughout the day to assuage hunger pangs during any
period of the diet.

*Interest value:*
Surprisingly high even on low Calorie (kilojoule) days, becoming more varied during the 1200 Calorie (5,040 kilojoule) mid-
phase. Menus are well balanced, based largely on fresh vegetables, salads, fruit, fish, poultry, lean meat, low fat cheeses,
wholemeal bread, cereals and pasta, baked potatoes and even
small amounts of jam (jelly), marmalade and cake (cookies).
Coffee, tea and herb teas or low salt bouillon drinks are also
permitted. For maximum flexibility there is a good selection of
alternative breakfast/lunch/dinner menus that may be
substituted at any time after the first fortnight of the diet or
used as a post diet weight maintenance plan. Vegetarians may
substitute pulses, seeds, nuts, grains for meat.

*Nutritional aspect:*
Because this diet involves only a few days of very restricted
Calorie (kilojoule) consumption and is based on a healthy
balance of protein, low fat, high fibre complex-carbohydrate
foods, with tremendous emphasis on fruit and vegetables, this
is certainly one of the better nutritionally thought-out slimming diets. Weight maintenance will obviously depend on
how closely you can stick to a diet of non-fattening foods.

**The Cambridge diet**
The most well-known and popular of the controversial, very

low Calorie (kilojoule) diets (VLCDs), the Cambridge Diet provides a mere 330 Calories (1,386 kilojoules) per day. This understandably allows dieters to achieve a degree of weight-reduction approaching that normally only seen as a result of near-starvation. Unlike other crash diets or fasting however, the meal replacements that form the basis of this diet have been formulated to provide all the vitamins, minerals and trace elements, as well as a supply of essential amino acids and fatty acids necessary for maintaining good health.

The selling point of the Cambridge Diet is that, despite providing a subsistence level of Calories (kilojoules), you will nevertheless still get all your nutritional requirements. For rapid and safe weight-loss, you simply substitute all normal meals with three liquid replacements or snack bars for four weeks only. Estimated weight-loss is initially around three to seven pounds (1.3–3 kg) per week. After this, a 400 Calorie (3,280 kilojoule) meal, which may be purchased ready-made from Cambridge Nutrition Limited, is added to the diet and you are supposed to juggle around with the meal replacements and low Calorie (kilojoule) meals until the target weight has been reached.

For anyone determined to lose a lot of surplus weight very quickly and safely, this is an ideal diet. It allows you to achieve an average weight-loss of 18 pounds (8 kg) in four weeks, and about 14 pounds (6kg) in each month thereafter.

According to Dr Alan Howard who devised the programme, far from being a fad diet, it was developed only after eight years of medical and nutritional research and stringent testing to establish its safety. Extensive monitoring of severely overweight people who have been on the Cambridge Diet for long periods suggest that side-effects are few, if any. Many advocates of the diet remark on feeling particularly well and enjoying high levels of energy, a fact which Dr Howard attributes to the improved quality of nutrition. Dieters often continue taking the various diet aids as a supplement with every-day food, even after their ideal weight has been reached.

The profit incentive method of marketing the Cambridge Diet has, however, aroused a certain amount of controversy. Only 'Cambridge Counsellors', men and women who have followed the diet themselves, are allowed to sell the product following a short period of training in the basic principles of nutrition. This they buy wholesale, and sell at a profit to other clients, keeping a percentage of the profit. Critics point out that, in spite of having little medical or nutritional background knowledge, counsellors are setting themselves up as diet experts and using hard-sell techniques to boost their profits.

Notwithstanding criticism, Cambridge counselling centres, most of them well run, are opening up throughout the country. They seem to offer valuable advice, encouragement and motivation for dieters.

**Verdict**
*Weight-loss potential:*
Excellent. Expect to lose about four pounds (2 kg), perhaps more, in a week and about one stone (6 kg) a month.
*Deprivation factor:*
Considerable. For four weeks you must take the Cambridge Diet three times a day, and eat no other food. You should also drink eight glasses of water, tea with lemon, and black coffee. Hunger is most nagging during the first three days, especially at night, but this wears off for most people towards the end of the first week of dieting. Eating out socially becomes very difficult on the Cambridge Diet, but on the other hand the meal replacements take all the planning out of eating to lose weight.
*Interest value:*
Very limited indeed. Boredom is a real problem since the basic 330 Calories (1,386 kilojoules) a day diet consists of liquid meal

replacements. There are also sweet-tasting meal bars, soups and a choice of four different 400-Calorie (3,280 kilojoule) slimming meals and desserts for those upping their Calorie (kilojoule) intake in the fifth week.

*Recommended for:*

Anyone really determined to lose a lot of weight fast, provided they do not eat out a lot, or enjoy a social life that revolves around eating and drinking. It is unsuitable for either breast-feeding or pregnant women or children. It is unlikely to inspire anyone hoping to change their eating habits for life. It seems a pointlessly punitive regime for those with merely seven or eight pounds (2.5–3.5 kg) to lose. People suffering from low energy levels and low blood sugar may find that tiredness, irritability, headaches or loss of energy can be a problem in the first few days, though this usually disappears after the first week.

*Nutritional aspect:*

VLCDs are rarely the answer for long-term weight control but like any slimming plan that restricts Calorie (kilojoule) intake they will reduce weight. With a VLCD most of the initial weight-loss is due to losses of body water and, despite manufacturer's reassurances, you could be losing more lean body tissue than is acceptable. As well as being potentially dangerous for some individuals VLCDs don't usually help to change eating habits, so weight is likely to be regained once you stop using them. But if you can maintain the loss by careful normal eating you'll get the best out of them.

On the positive side, VLCDs are a better and safer way to achieve a quick weight-loss than total fasting.

### Herbalife

A 1,000-Calories (4,200 kilojoules)-a-day diet based on meal replacements taken in the form of high protein/low fat powder mixed with fruit juice or milk. The diet is claimed by manufacturers to be based on vitamins, minerals and 'nutritional herbs' needed to promote good health and prevent hunger or loss of energy. Herbalife meal replacements are distributed via a self-propagating chain of distributors, on similar lines to the Cambridge Diet. Weight-loss is not as rapid as with the VLCD.

**Univite**

Based on similar lines to the Cambridge Diet, Univite offer the choice of ten 100-Calorie (420 kilojoule) meal replacements which are taken whisked with hot or cold water to provide 330 Calories (1,386 kilojoules) a day. The manufacturers claim the product has all the recommended daily allowances of vitamins, minerals, trace elements and electrolytes necessary for good health. The diet can be taken for three weeks as the sole source of nutrition, but low Calorie (kilojoule) meals must be added in the fourth week. Distribution is via a nationwide network of 'advisors' as with the Cambridge Diet and Herbalife systems. The cost works out as more expensive than buying, for example, other brands in chemists or drugstores. Weight-loss potential is considerable, averaging approximately 14 to 16 pounds (6–7 kg) in one month.

**The VLCD debate**

Although they are currently fashionable, there is nothing new about today's very low Calorie (kilojoule) diets (VLCDs) such as the Cambridge Diet and Univite. They are simply another variation on semi-fasting regimes and crash diets. These have long been popular because of their ability to induce rapid weight reduction, but now they are put across with all the hype of modern marketing techniques. Yet there is one little difference: the various manufacturers claim that these diets, in spite of their low calorific value, are far safer because they contain all the nutrients necessary for good health.

Certainly the number of satisfied, and apparently healthy, slimmers who have lost weight on VLCDs testifies to their efficacy as well their safety. While eating nothing but grape-fruit and eggs may cause you to lose as much weight in a fortnight as say the Cambridge Diet, you will probably derive better nutrition, and, say the manufacturers, feel healthy and more energetic, if you opt for the 'all-in' VLCD. They also claim that one of the main reasons slimmers give up stringent diets is because these offer an insufficiently high level of all-round nutrition leading to tiredness, irritability, lack of energy, dizziness and other typical slimmers' complaints.

VLCDs have been widely used with excellent results in obesity clinics attached to major hospitals throughout the country. Stringent dieting under medical supervision is one thing, but doing it alone is quite another. Some doctors, therefore, express concern that staying on a VLCD for too long can lead to excessive loss of lean body tissue. This may harm the vital organs, including the heart, with the risk of severe illness or even death. Manufacturers of VLCDs stress, therefore, that no one should embark on such a diet without first consulting their doctor, and that periods of taking low Calorie (kilojoule) meal replacements as sole source of nutrition *must* be interrupted regularly by the intake of more Calories (kilojoules), and reintroduction of a more balanced diet.

Sensationalist reports from America of deaths caused by following VLCDs are needlessly alarmist. They are due to misleading or incomplete information about the modern VLCDs. In the 1970s the infamous liquid protein diets, allegedly to blame for a number of deaths, were in fact composed of collagen, an inferior grade protein. They contained insufficient essential nutrients, such as selenium to maintain the necessary electrolyte balance to regulate heart function. Although numbers of people in America are reported to have died on the Cambridge Diet (not the same formula as the British Cambridge Diet) the American FDA has never positively attributed these deaths to the diet. There is some evidence that drug and alcohol abuse, and existing ill-health, may have been predisposing factors.

Another area of concern is the relative protein value of VLCDs. Adequate intake of protein is essential for the regular maintenance and repair of vital body organs. So how much protein do we need to stay healthy? The World Health Organisation says 1.5 oz (37 g) a day. The Cambridge Diet provides 1.2 oz (33 g), Univite 1.55 oz (42 g). Univite also advise anyone worried about adequate protein intake to add just 1 oz (25 g) of powdered skimmed milk to their liquid meals or coffee, to boost protein levels by another 0.3 oz (9 g) without affecting the rate of weight-loss.

Although many people have slimmed successfully using VLCDs, at the time of writing at least one major enquiry is taking place to determine whether they should remain available on the market in their present form. It is unlikely, in the light of their good safety record, that commercial VLCDs will be banned outright, although some doctors would like their Calorie (kilojoule) content to be raised to a more acceptable 600 or 800 Calories (2,520 or 3,360 kilojoules).

# – 2 –
# Dietary Alternatives and Slimming Aids

A tremendous amount of confusion surrounds the whole terminology of slimming. The word 'slimming' itself, which, when used commercially, carries highly emotive and suggestive overtones, is consistently misinterpreted by those eager to lose weight. At the same time, it is regularly, and often quite deliberately, misused by manufacturers of foods, drugs and appliances geared to the ever-burgeoning 'slimmers' market. In America, the sales figures for special slimmer's foods and aids has reached staggering proportions, with an estimated five billion dollars spent each year collectively by men and women in the attempt to lose weight. According to one US supermarket chain, sales of low calorie foods and prepackaged slimmers' meals have been rising by 15 per cent annually over the past five years while sugar-free 'diet' sodas and other soft drinks now account for one-fifth of the nation's soft drinks sales. A crucial point, so often conveniently overlooked in our search for an easy way to lose weight, is that there is no substitute for self-control. Therefore there is no *product* – as yet, at any rate – which can make you lose weight.

Strictly speaking, then, the term 'slimming product' is a misnomer, since we can only become slimmer through eating fewer Calories (kilojoules) or burning up a greater number – or both. Despite recent attempts to crack down on the number of misleading advertising claims made by manufacturers of dietary and slimming aids by imposing new and stricter rules, when you glance through any glossy magazine or popular newspaper, the success with which many advertisers continue to flout these rules, or circumvent them, is glaringly evident.

Whether dietary aids can in fact help someone who is trying to reduce weight do so more easily or rapidly depends on each individual concerned, as well as on their personal expectations. For example, there is no argument that replacing sugar with saccharine in a cup of tea does reduce its Calorific (kilojoule) value virtually to nil. This makes low-Calorie (kilojoule) sweeteners good news for anyone hooked on vast quantities of sweet beverages. Eating twice as many slices of low-Calorie (kilojoule) crispbread or 'slimmers' bread to assuage hunger ensures, however, that your Calorie (kilojoule) intake is the same as if you'd eaten ordinary bread. Similarly, eating a meal-replacement snack bar at teatime as well as for the lunch or dinner it was designed to replace, means you take in extra Calories (kilojoules) rather than limiting them.

Many dieters come to rely on the security and ease of prepackaged meal replacement products. Their Calorie (kilojoule) content is clearly stated, taking the guesswork out of Calorie (kilojoule) – counting and the decision-making out of meal-planning. But such products may prove an expensive way to slim in the long run (many slimmers also find them unacceptably bland or tasteless). It is worth remembering that these are no more filling, nutritious, tasty or non-fattening than the well thought-out meal replacements you can prepare at home. Eating diced raw vegetables or munching a few spoons of bran will fill you up or take the edge off your appetite as effectively as any commercial product, if not more so. It is certainly cheaper. The difference lies in convenience.

Slimmers leading a very busy life, perhaps working away from home all day, may understandably opt for the ease and lack of fuss of a prepackaged slimmers' snack or meal-substitute.

When it comes to prescription drugs such as diuretics, hormone extracts and those designed to speed up metabolism as an aid to weight-loss, the whole question of what is suitable – and more important, safe – is far more clear-cut. All such drugs, which basically interfere with the synchronisation and rhythm of fundamental bodily functions, are potentially hazardous: they may cause unpleasant and dangerous side-effects, while also posing the risk of addiction. Drugs to aid weight-reduction are suitable only under special circumstances for a limited number of people who are chronically overweight. They must be prescribed by a qualified and experienced doctor who is familiar with the patient's medical history. Judicious prescribing is the keynote here.

Drugs to help weight-loss can only be taken over a limited period and the patient's progress and physical health must be regularly monitored. Once again, it is vital to stress that no reputable or responsible doctor will prescribe drugs to assist weight reduction without also recommending a suitably healthy, balanced, low-Calorie (kilojoule) diet. Drugs alone will not have the effect of causing weight-loss.

Never accept slimming pills from friends, acquaintances or unqualified practitioners, especially if you are not sure what they are. A quick consultation with your local pharmacist should cast light on the nature of any unidentified 'slimming pills' you might be tempted to take. Vitamin manufacturers and healthfood shops have been trading in so-called 'safe' slimmers' aids for decades, if not centuries. The only difference between the traditional nostrums touted by old-style herbalists and those sold by today's modern emporia is the pseudo-scientific sales jargon and sophisticated packaging.

The numerous teas, tonics, herbs, minerals, vitamins and 'organic' nutrients alledged to promote weight-loss will certianly do you no harm. There is no significant evidence that they work, either, which is why I have not singled them out in this review.

## DIETARY ALTERNATIVES AND SLIMMING AIDS – AN A–Z

### Artificial sweeteners
*Saccharin and aspartame*
Saccharin is probably the best-known artificial sweetener of all. It is 300 times as sweet as sugar but leaves a slightly bitter aftertaste. Although massive doses have been shown to cause cancer in animals, the amounts normally used in coffee or tea are so low that risks to health have been ruled out.

A more recent arrival on the sweeteners market is made from aspartame, a combination of two amino acids which is about 180 times as sweet as sugar but tastes very similar to the real thing and has none of the metallic or bitter aftertaste of saccharin. When used in combination with saccharin, as in certain low-Calorie (kilojoule) soft diet drinks, it masks the taste of saccharin. Unfortunately, unlike saccharin, aspartame cannot be used for cooking because it breaks down under prolonged and high heat.

Since one teaspoon (5 ml) of sugar contains about 20 Calories (84 kilojoules), artificial sweeteners, which contain no Calories (kilojoules) at all, are a useful replacement for ordinary sugar in tea or coffee and as an alternative sweetening agent for cereals and desserts. A really heavy tea or coffee-drinker could save as much as 3,500 Calories (14.7 megajoules) a week, simply by replacing sugar with a sweetener! Many zero-Calorie (kilojoule) diet drinks (e.g. Diet Pepsi) are based on these substitutes. Although swapping sugar for artificial sweeteners will help cut down Calories (kilojoules), it will of course do nothing to curb a 'sweet tooth', since this can only be achieved by limiting the amount of sweet-tasting foods and drinks in the diet.

**Appetite suppressants**
Taken about half an hour before a meal, ideally these products should help you to eat less by reducing hunger. Slimming cubes contain liquid glucose. They have a chewy texture, come in different flavours, and work on the theory that if you raise your blood sugar level before a meal you will not feel like eating as much as usual. There is no reason why these, rather than any other sweet-tasting snack, should reduce appetite, and in many cases no effects are experienced whatsoever. Indeed, you might end up eating the cubes and immediately afterwards tucking into your normal meal as usual, thereby actually upping your Calorie (kilojoule) intake!

Bran tablets sold in chemist's, and drugstores as a slimming aid, should be eaten ten minutes before meals. Bran is 63 per cent indigestible cellulose and these tablets are meant to impart a feeling of fullness when eaten before a meal. A number of meal 'substitutes' contain a high percentage of bran to counteract the problem of hunger pangs that linger after eating low-Calorie (kilojoule) food. 'Bulk fillers' are usually based on an indigestible substance called methylcellulose. When eaten, this swells up and expands in the stomach, thereby supposedly reducing appetite.

These appetite-suppressants may work better for some slimmers than for others. Certain people find their filling action wears off after a few weeks, as their system become more dependent on the substance. The main drawbacks of these tablets are that they have a laxative action and can also cause flatulence, distension and stomach cramp. Eating a piece of wholemeal bread or a few spoonfuls of bran is just as likely to blunt the appetite. Slimmers' chewing gum is a sweet chewing gum spiked with benzocaine, a harmless mild anaesthetic, which temporarily takes the edge off your appetite. However, it is more likely to briefly take the edge off your sense of taste than to have any lasting impact on your desire for food.

## Diuretics

Mild diuretics based on herbal extracts or caffeine sold without prescription in chemist's, drugstores and healthfood shops are a safe method of controlling fluid retention, especially when associated with the premenstrual syndrome.

Herbal extracts such as dandelion, burdock and sarsaparilla are just some of the natural substances known for their supposed harmless diuretic properties which are sold as an aid to overcome fluid retention. There is, however, no evidence that any of these preparations can help to reduce weight.

Prescription diuretics are usually prescribed for patients with glaucoma, lung, heart, kidney or liver disorders which result in excessive retention of fluid in the body. These drugs work by suppressing the re-absorption of salt from the urine back into the bloodstream, thereby encouraging greater elimination of salt and water from the body. Continued and prolonged use can cause excessive salt and water loss. This in turn leads to a fall in vital minerals and trace elements, including potassium and calcium, which can prove a serious health hazard.

Other side-effects of taking diuretics include nausea, dizziness, diarrhoea, numbness, skin rashes, sensitivity of the skin to sunlight, thirst and loss of appetite – which in turn leads to further depletion of minerals and other nutrients.

Diuretics are strictly bad news when it comes to weight-loss. Unfortunately, they are still commonly prescribed by many unscrupulous so-called 'slimming doctors' and weight-loss clinics. They are responsible for perpetuating the myth that loss of weight always equals loss of fat, when in fact it is often solely due to elimination of fluid. The really scary thing about the constant use of diuretics is that they are ultimately self-defeating; if water is forced quickly out of the body it is re-absorbed even faster. Upsetting the body's delicate chemistry for maintaining and regulating fluid level results in chronic fluid retention. This explains why many slimmers taking diuretics experience constant weight-gain following reduction, and eventually become hooked on the drug.

--------------- *DANGERS OF DEHYDRATION* ---------------

Apart from the risk of addiction, the inevitable result of taking strong diuretics over a long period is that the body becomes severely dehydrated, with the risk of eventual heart and kidney failure. Being on a severely restricted diet and taking diuretics is in itself a prescription for disaster, since slimming diets often tend to lead to deficiencies in essential minerals, including selenium, zinc, magnesium and potassium. Taking diuretics flushes these out of the body even faster.

Another category of people particularly at risk are those with bulimia (the compulsive binge/starve syndrome). When someone who has been near to starvation and become deficient in these minerals then overeats, the heart and other vital organs may be placed under undue stress. The lack of adequate resources can lead to serious illness.

Other 'natural' diuretics that are far less harmful are drinks based on a group of substances called xanthines which include caffeine, theophylline and theobromine. Present in tea, coffee, cola and cocoa, their mild diuretic effect is caused by increasing the rate of salt excretion through urination, without risk of serious side-effects. Drinking too much strong coffee or tea, however, can crank up the body's production of stress hormones, causing irritability, nervous tension, sleeplessness, headaches and shaking and is therefore not recommended for anyone with hypertension.

## Meal replacements

So called 'slimming foods' constitute far and away the greatest money-spinner within the slimming industry. The sale of ever-proliferating low-Calorie (kilojoule) snack bars, chocolate or candy bars, soups, crispbread, rolls, cereals and replacement foods makes up a very large proportion of any chemist's or drugstore's turnover. These prepackaged replacement foods, whose Calorie (kilojoule) content is usually clearly displayed, are ideal for slimmers who not only want the guesswork taken out of Calorie (kilojoule) counting, but also cannot be bothered, or are too busy, to prepare their own nonfattening meals. Some meal replacements today aspire to cordon bleu status, and special low-Calorie (kilojoule) meals available in supermarkets are inventive, tasty and of the highest possible quality.

Eating low-Calorie (kilojoule) foods, therefore, does not condemn you to making do with a poor imitation of the original. However, it does mean you end up paying more money to eat fewer Calories (kilojoules), so this is not a cost-effective way to slim. And if your goal is permanent weight-reduction, it is to your advantage to learn to plan and prepare low-Calorie (kilojoule) meals at home, since any successful dietary modifications are those adhered to for long periods, or indeed for life.

Special slimmers' biscuit or cookie meals provide an excellent alternative to say, the filling but fattening sandwich you might normally have for lunch or the gooey mid-morning or teatime fattening snack. Not only are these sweet and savoury biscuits or cookies low in Calories (kilojoules), but they may contain methycellulose or bran to fill you up faster. The same goes for slimmers' crunchy nut and chocolate bars, a tasty alternative to the fattening chocolate or candy snacks.

Slimmers' drinks constitute a meal in a glass that is often mixed with milk and which tastes like a milk shake. These can satisfy your craving for sweet-tasting foods. They are usually sold in packs designed to provide a very low-Calorie (kilojoule) daily eating plan (i.e. under 500 Calories (2,100 kilojoules)), if used as a sole source of nutrition. The problem with these liquid meals is that they tend to taste bland and unnatural, and using them for too long as substitutes for proper food becomes boring. The lack of roughage may cause constipation.

If taken as a sole source of nutrition for too long without medical guidance, staying on a very low-Calorie (kilojoule) diet poses a risk of ill-health through malnutrition. Nor does it help alter eating habits in the long run.

Low-fat cottage cheese or ricotta, skimmed milk and low-Calorie (kilojoule) crispbread, will all help slimmers reduce Calorie (kilojoule) intake. Slimming breads have weight for weight exactly the same Calorie (kilojoule) content as ordinary bread – they are simply cut in thinner slices and contain more air. Low fat spreads dilute margarine or butter with water and therefore contain 50 per cent fewer Calories (kilojoules). Skimmed milk and skimmed milk powders also have half the Calories (kilojoules) of full fat milk. Low fat versions of salad dressing and mock ice cream desserts also provide a low-Calorie (kilojoule) option to the real thing.

When used regularly in place of full high fat or high sugar products, all these slimmers' alternatives can help considerably in lowering daily Calorie (kilojoule) intake.

## HCG (Human Chorionic Gonadotrophin)

HCG was first introduced in the early 1950s by Dr A T W Simeons, a slimming doctor based in Rome, who claimed that

HCG, a pregnancy hormone extract, can 'mobilise' accumulated stores of fat by causing it to be burned off as fuel. Fat is allegedly lost 'selectively', from those parts of the body where superfluous inches are concentrated, for instance, the thighs and waist, but not the face.

The treatment consists of a minimum of 21 injections, backed up by a rigid 500-Calories (2,100 kilojoules) per day diet. For weight-loss of over 15 pounds (7 kg), the course is a maximum of 40 injections, followed by a mandatory break of six weeks. After the course is finished patients must avoid all starches for three weeks until the new weight has stabilised to within two pounds (900 g) of the weight on completion of the course.

Reports of the success of HCG in promoting weight-loss are purely anecdotal and there is absolutely no evidence to corroborate claims that HCG can 'burn off' fat. It is, of course, hardly surprising that slimmers *do* lose weight on the treatment – as would anybody on a 500-Calories (120 kilojoules) diet. The crux of the matter is, are the injections a contributory factor? The answer is, probably not.

### Weight-reducing drugs

These drugs have been widely criticised as having little place in the treatment of obesity, since possible benefits are largely outweighed by risks involved.

All slimming drugs work basically in the same way, affecting that part of the brain which controls appetite and generally 'speeding up' bodily function. However, some are safer than others and formulations as well as side-effects vary. Amphetamine, the earliest of all appetite suppressors, is highly addictive and in its pure, original form is now rarely prescribed because of dangerous side-effects. So-called 'safe' amphetamines or amphetamine compounds are now more frequently prescribed for very overweight or chronically obese people, because they have a less stimulating effect on the heart and circulation. The most widely used of these compounds is Diethylpropion. This initially reduces appetite, although the effect tends to wear off after some weeks, causing a very real risk of dependence if the dose is increased. For this reason, such drugs are unsuitable for long-term use, and should only be prescribed intermittently as a form of on/off therapy for people with a serious weight problem.

*Drawbacks of drugs*
Addiction, with the attendant risks to general health, is what worries doctors most about these drugs. There is also the fact that taking them may prevent you from eating as much as you would normally, but for a limited period only, and your long-term eating habits will remain unchanged. Much the same goes for other slimming drugs. All have a very limited potential in controlling appetite and are no substitute for will-power or a change in eating patterns.

The general consensus of opinion amongst doctors is that these drugs should only be prescribed for a limited period under specific circumstances, as for example where there is a real risk to health due to obesity.

*Slimming clinics and dolly mixtures*
Beware of unscrupulous self-styled slimming 'clinics' which often hand out a selection of unidentified pills to unsuspecting clients as an aid to so-called 'dynamic weight-loss'. Don't let the jargon or sales talk confuse or mislead you. Pills with a 'thermogenic' or 'thermodynamic' action, which supposedly mobilise fat stores through 'stimulus of catecholamines' (natural adrenalin) are, in plain language, no more – or rather no less – than amphetamines or related compounds. Worse still, a number of slimming centres have been known to supply dieters with a dangerous dolly mixture of pills includ-

ing diuretics, amphetamine-like drugs and thyroid extracts, while recommending a very low-Calorie (kilojoule) diet.

The net effect of subjecting yourself to such an assault course could well be that you undermine your health and put your body into a state of shock, with extremely severe ill-effects. And even if your health is not seriously affected, the chances of reducing weight for a significant period are minimal.

### Thyroid hormones

Thyroxine and Tri-iodthyroxine are secreted by the thyroid gland and help to regulate growth and metabolism. The use of thyroid hormones to treat obese patients was a fairly common practice over 20 years ago, but has fallen from favour because of dangerous side-effects. The problem is that only large doses work in helping to reduce weight, especially in the case of chronically obese people, and this is harmful to health.

However, doctors at Addenbrookes Hospital in Cambridge, England, have found that giving small amounts of TA3, a by-product of Thyroxine, can help certain individuals already on a weight reducing diet to overcome the 'plateau stage'. This is the term given to the stage in a weight-loss programme when a lower metabolic rate radically slows down weight-loss to about half of what it was at the beginning of a diet. TA3 can help to raise the metabolic rate again, leading to further necessary weight-loss. However, very obese people are generally resistant to these modest doses of thyroid hormone.

People having thyroid treatment, who only want to lose a small amount of weight fairly quickly, run the risk of losing a large amount of protein from the body. In the long run this could prove dangerous, as well as upsetting the complex and delicate mechanism of the thyroid gland.

# – 3 –
# *Salon Treatments*

The slimming and beauty industries, both closely allied, have been spawned by a growth in body consciousness sometimes bordering on the obsessive. Together they represent an area of phenomenally rapid commercial growth. Rising profits reflect a burgeoning consumer market, eager to slim down and shape up, whatever the financial cost.

The fact that claims in the slimming/beauty business range from the legitimate to the ludicrous does little to deter the slimming and fitness enthusiast from investing in bodily improvement, largely on spec. But while it is tempting to regard the beauty industry overall as a con, deriving profits from the blatant exploitation of a woman's hopes and insecurities about her self-image, such a summary dismissal would be as unhelpful as it is blinkered. Some, though by no means all, salon treatments do offer *certain* women (and it is women, not men who constitute the major proportion of salon clients and health club members) a chance of improving *some* figure problems. Just how much and which type of improvement salon treatment can deliver depends on the individual woman concerned, and her particular problem.

The criteria by which different women choose and ultimately judge such treatments vary considerably. Few salons with any respectable reputation would claim to be able to do much for the chronically overweight or those with gross associated figure defects.

## Treatment for figure problems

However, that still leaves a large proportion of women whose physical proportions fall far short of what they regard as ideal. Rare is the woman who is happy with her shape. Women of normal or near-normal weight often have a relatively slim and firm, well-proportioned body but want to overcome one or two isolated figure problems. Such problems may be inherited or else have developed as a result of ageing, child-bearing or ill health. The most common amongst these are sagging breasts, flabby tummy and, above all, superflous hard or lumpy fat and puckered skin on thighs, buttocks, hips, the notorious 'saddle bags' or 'riding breech bulges' – commonly known in the beauty business as cellulite.

## Anorexic or overweight?

Obsessive nit-picking over physical shape is commonest amongst the slim and good-looking. Many girls and young women of seemingly near-perfect, model girl proportions will consult a salon for treatment of a defect so minor and unnoticeable that some beauticians may even refuse to carry out treatment. Often suffering from a distorted self-image, they may confuse the issue of weight and shape and can be in danger of developing the slimmer's disease anorexia nervosa.

In contrast, other women with obvious excess weight problems, who are also chronically unfit, may visit a beauty therapist to obtain advice on diet and exercise. By undergoing a programme of salon treatments they may find added incentive to continue losing weight and exercising as a result of encouragement from their beautician, besides certain visible cosmetic improvements that result from treatment. Not for nothing do many beauticians adopt the role of confidante or psychotherapist. The motivation gained as a result of having one's health, body and figure problems sympathetically analysed, discussed and treated, can prove of inestimable value to a women who for years has abused her looks and neglected her body.

Salon treatments are, it must be said, no substitute for dieting or exercise, but in certain cases they can help to improve figure problems. The more specific your individual problem, the easier it is to evaluate the mode of treatment available for the disorder in question, and assess how successfully it might help your condition, if at all. Knowing what is and isn't possible in purely physiological terms, can, however, help cut down on disappointment and save wasted money.

## Caution: breasts and tummy, claims that stretch the imagination

Misleading claims are still made by many manufacturers for spot slimming products, i.e. products which treat one specific area. Thankfully, advertising codes of practice are somewhat stricter today than a few years ago, although in the opinion of most doctors the rules which cover advertising and marketing are not strict enough. There is, for example, no known serum, cream, oil, machine, body wrap, corrective bra, or other gadget which can reduce outsize or firm sagging breasts. Breasts are made up of fatty and glandular tissue and skin, hence their shape and tilt can only be altered through surgery. Yet products which purport to be able to 'tighten', 'lift', 'firm', 'reform' and 'dissolve the fatty tissues' of drooping and excessively large breasts, still proliferate in shops and salons.

### SUPPORT FOR EXERCISE

Certain types of exercise, such as swimming and weight lifting, may help to firm the muscles which surround the breasts, so helping to support breast tissue which is still relatively young and firm. Wearing a well-designed supporting bra, especially while exercising, can help prevent premature sagging of breast tissue. Women with heavy breasts often find that bra straps cut in and cause excessive discomfort. They can now exercise with greater ease by wearing one of the new exercise bras, fashioned rather like the upper section of a sleeveless leotard.

The effects of extreme weight changes, child-bearing, breast-feeding and the ageing process in general, however, all militate against any woman except for those with very small breasts escaping the eventual downward pull of gravity which distends once-firm connective tissues and surface skin.

Treatments that claim to tighten loose skin on tummy or breasts that is scarred by stretchmarks should also be dismissed as so much hokum. Whatever the ads say, once the connective tissues and epidermis have been over-stretched and scars have appeared, no amount of massage with oils and serums can mend ruptured collagen, the protein in the tissues responsible for maintaining the skin's smoothness and resilience. On the other hand, the livid red colour of many fresh scars and stretchmarks can be partially faded to a less noticeable silvery colour by keeping the skin moisturised and supple with the use of a good quality body oil or cream.

---

## APPLES AND PEARS

Inevitably, given today's emphasis on androgynous fashion, featuring figure-hugging, all-revealing sportswear, jeans, tailored trousers, second-skin exercise garments, nude look swimsuits and underwear, 'lower body reshaping' is the most lucrative area of treatment for most salons. Today's sexy, long-stemmed female ideal with her slender thighs, narrow hips, flat small bottom, as represented by fashion and media alike, is an almost impossible model of female perfection for the average well rounded, curvy-hipped woman of 5 ft 2 in (1.5 m) to live up to.

Many of today's fashions seem specifically designed for an impossibly glamorous and perfect 'super woman', pursuing a fantasy lifestyle. What's more, hers is a look that is almost impossible to fake. This is because unlike earlier, more elaborate fashions, today's minimalist styles are cruelly body exposing. They allow little opportunity for the concealment of physical defects. Little wonder, therefore, that you can't be a successful follower of current fashion, be it at the beach in g-string bikin bottom, or partying in clinging crêpe catsuit, if you have a dropped, wobbly bottom or bulging thighs!

**Mysterious cellulite**

According to the market laws of supply and demand, anti-cellulite treatments have become potentially the biggest money-spinners – even though no one knows exactly what cellulite really is and if it exists at all! For example, does cellulite have certain characteristics that distinguish it from other types of fat? According to doctors, fat is fat wherever it lodges and those saddle bags and other bulges of hard or corrugated-looking excess tissue on hips, legs and bottom are no exception.

But then why is it that a woman may diet and exercise until she has reached her normal weight or be naturally slim, even underweight, yet still suffer from a heavy or outsize bottom and superfluous flesh on the thighs, while other areas above the waist may by comparison appear quite scrawny? Scientists trying to unravel the quirks of fat distribution have come up with quite a plausible theory. Fat build-up seems to be dictated by the ratio between two types of receptors on the surface of fat cells: Beta-1 receptors, which stimulate fat breakdown, and the Alpha-2 variety which inhibit its loss. Women generally tend to carry extra fatty tissue around the hips, thighs and buttocks. Much of this is made up of fat-retaining Alpha receptors, explaining that widespread phenomenon, the female 'pear' shape, while men have more on their stomach giving them a pot-bellied 'apple' shape.

### Losing weight and staying the same

Weight-loss often does little to alter the fundamental distribution of body fat. Men who lose weight may simply become less rotund 'apples' and women slim down to smaller 'pears', slimmer above the waist, still bulky below. Although extra abdominal fat is regarded as a greater health hazard than pelvic fat because of its correlation to an increased risk of heart disease and diabetes, this is of little consolation to the split-sized woman.

### Like mother, like daughter

Fat distribution is very largely inherited. The so-called British 'pear' shape is no more endemic amongst British women than it is amongst those of the rest of Europe, the Middle and Far East, South and North America. Therefore, the tendency to develop large thighs may be passed down along generations of females within a family.

### Female fat vs. male fat

There is also some research to suggest that, apart from being unevenly distributed, female and male tissue also differs in the way it is laid down. Female surface skin is thinner than that of a man and therefore more likely to reveal any bulging, superfluous fatty deposits underneath. The connective fibres which divide up female fat tissue and hold it in place tend to be laid down in an irregular pattern. This pushes the fat into large round uneven globules, creating the familiar spongy 'mattress' effect when pinched, and making the surface skin look dimpled and marbled. In contrast, the individual fibres of men's fatty tissue have a lattice-like weave which allows the tissues to expand and contract when weight is lost, giving a smoother overall effect. Even in cases of excessive surplus fat, the tissue is arranged into neater symmetrical units which hold it all into a smoother shape.

Most beauty therapists, however, claim that the lumpy, bumpy, adhesive quality that distinguishes cellulite from the smooth uniform fat on neighbouring tummy, waist, arms, etc, is caused primarily by an accumulation of fluid and toxic waste. This, they believe, has become trapped within the fatty tissues, largely through impaired, sluggish circulation and faulty lymphatic drainage. This is attributable to factors as diverse as stress, faulty diet, poor posture, lack of exercise and hormonal imbalance.

**Cellulite is bunk, says doctors**
According to the medical profession, all this is bunk – and so are the treatments. Claims that certain machines, injections or forms of massage can 'melt away' surplus tissue or 'burn up' excess fat cells or 'unlock and release trapped toxins and fat' have neither rational foundation nor scientific credibility.

**Beauty therapists undeterred**
Meanwhile, the beauty profession remains resolutely undeterred by what they dismiss as medical scepticism and a stony indifference on the part of doctors to what is, for many women, a very real and upsetting psychological problem.

The primary aims of all current anti-cellulite treatments are therefore based on stimulating circulation, counteracting fluid-retention, softening, breaking up and redistributing uneven build-up of hard, lump, diet-resistant fat. The credibility of these treatments varies greatly. The truth is that there are a number of well-tried and tested treatments, some of which have been around for a number of years. According to reports from reputable and experienced therapists, *and* a fair percentage of satisfied clients, these said treatments do seem to succeed in improving certain localised figure problems to some extent.

## Treatment for cellulite

Localised reshaping, or spot reduction treatments, rarely work well on their own. It is well acknowledged in the salon business that those therapists who obtain the best results in reshaping and reducing stubborn, localised fat often do so through insisting their clients adhere to a sensible eating pattern, and take some form of regular exercise, while undergoing intensive regular, and sometimes long-term, treatment.

Clients who expect to see instant, visible improvements in their figure must inevitably be disappointed. As with dieting or with exercising, the key to success lies in committed self-discipline. Experimenting with just a couple of trial sessions of any figure treatment or undergoing a course or programme in a desultory, uncommitted fashion – one session here and there with long gaps in between – is a waste of time and money. It is almost certainly guaranteed to produce no significant results, even in the case of minor figure problems.

## Tightening-up

Most beauty therapists subscribe to the old adage that correct weight does not necessarily equal a correct figure. Hence the emphasis in all treatments is to tighten, recontour and try to reduce inches (centimetres), rather than pounds (kilos). Using a tape measure to assess the measurements of different parts of the body before, during, and after a course of treatment can prove misleading, since it is difficult to take measurements at the identical part of the body each time. A far better way to gauge whether you are beginning to shape up or not is to wear a very tight pair of trousers or skirt before embarking on a course of treatment. Assess your overall contours according to how tightly or loosely the garment fits as the treatment progresses.

The actual degree of improvement, how many inches (centimetres), if any, are lost, how much sleeker, tauter, less bulky or dimpled and generally streamlined, say, the thighs or waist become and for how long these effects last, depends on many factors. These include how many treatments are involved, individual physical type, age, how close you are to your target weight, and general lifestyle.

Broadly speaking, a woman of normal weight in her twenties or thirties who eats a well-balanced, non-fattening diet and takes regular exercise, but has excess flesh on the upper thighs, will tend to notice more rapid improvements than a woman in her mid to late forties or fifties with more extensive figure problems, who is perhaps slightly overweight and has a sedentary lifestyle.

------------------------ *WHAT'S AVAILABLE* ------------------------

## Massage

The world's oldest therapy is as popular today as it was amongst the ancient civilisations of Greece, Rome and Egypt. Only these days, what's on offer is a comprehensive range of methods, from classical Swedish techniques and high-tech electronic systems, to centuries-old, esoteric oriental methods of healing.

Massage used on its own will not directly slim or reshape the body. Its principle benefits lie in relaxing mind and body, soothing and unknotting tense muscles, relieving strain and pain, stimulating sluggish circulation, and encouraging the flow of lymph fluids. So, if you follow the premise that the root cause of cellulite is often sluggish circulation, fluid retention, impaired lymph drainage and congestion of the tissues, then it follows that, indirectly, massage can help. It can stop fluid retention, counteract puffy swollen tissues, especially on the legs, and soften and smooth the surface tissues.

*Vigorous shape-up*
There are also a number of specialised 'recontouring' techniques used by certain therapists, specifically to soften and break up areas of hard superfluous fat on arms, waist, hips, thighs, bottom. For anyone expecting a gentle and soothing massage it is important to point out that these are vigorous, even aggressive in the extreme.

**CTM (Connective Tissue Massage)**
Consists of intensive kneading, pinching, knuckling, wringing movements over areas of surplus flesh which is lifted, twisted, rolled and pushed up almost to the bone in an attempt to break up hard, adhesive fat and flatten lumpy contours.

Intensity of treatment depends very much on individual discomfort thresholds, which usually rise as treatments progress. Well-trained therapists always take care not to cause pain or unattractive, uncomfortable bruising. For anyone suffering from varicose veins or broken capillaries, this form of leg and thigh massage must be tempered according to the condition.

**Lymphatic drainage**
This form of massage is often combined with CTM in cases of cellulite and fluid retention, to decongest the tissues and aid elimination of surplus fluid. In contrast to CTM, lymphatic drainage is based on slow, long stroking, raking or combing movements along the superficial lymphatic vessels to stimulate the flow of tissue fluids. Massage is concentrated around

one area at a time and the slow, regular rhythm and broad, sweeping strokes used make this a deeply relaxing treatment.

## Aromatherapy

This combines the use of pure, therapeutic plant extracts or 'essential oils' with a variety of different massage techniques to decongest the tissues, aid lymphatic drainage and stimulate circulation. According to practitioners, these various plant oils have many therapeutic properties and act on the body both by inhalation, as well as through penetration of the upper layers of the skin.

## Shiatsu and acupressure

These are the two main oriental forms of massage. They are based on stimulating the body's acupressure points to boost circulation and relax or strengthen the various organs and systems. They are often referred to as acupuncture without needles. Pressure varies from mild to very strong and is usually exerted with the edges of thumb and fingers, although some therapists may use the knuckles, knees and even their feet to obtain the necessary pressure.

## Electronic alternatives

Most top therapists agree that when it comes to giving a vigorous and deeply probing massage, there is no electronic method equal to a strong pair of hands. The trouble is that a really strong pair of hands, capable of giving a first-class massage, is not that easy to find purely on spec. Those masseurs who seem to obtain the best results using connective tissue massage and other forms of hand massage are recognised principally for their ability to probe, grip, lift and manipulate superfluous flesh, even on those parts of the body which are fiddly and difficult to get at – the inner thigh, around the knees, crease line and buttock overhang.

By comparison, massage machines offer the practitioner an easier alternative since they can be switched on and left to do all the heavy duty work. The problem with many massage machines is that they can only be used up and down or across large surfaces of the body, and although the speed of the vibrations can be decreased and increased, the depth of massage is less simple to alter.

Altogether, fingers are more adaptable and give a deeper massage than electronic equipment. However, many salons sensibly use *both*, alternating between mechanical and manual massage during the course of one session. For example, one top salon, well known for its very successful 'bottom-lifting' and firming treatments and anti-cellulite courses, combines half an hour's deep power vibratory massage with another half hour's deep manual massage, both of these interspersed with a further half hour's treatment with an electronic exercise machine and the application of warm poultices. All this adds up to a very intensive two-and-a-half-hour treatment which, very sensibly, the salon insists must be taken on four consecutive days followed by four days alternating with rest days, on the principle that treatment must be intensive and vigorous in order to obtain the desired effects.

*Two types of massage machines*

There are two principle types of massage equipment; vibratory and suction. The most widely used and well-known vibratory massage unit is the G5, standard equipment at most beauty salons as well as osteopathy and physiotherapy clinics. The steady rhythm of electronic vibratory massage is deeply relaxing and works well to soothe tight, tense muscles, rev up circulation etc. Opinion as to how well it breaks up cellulite varies from practitioner to practitioner.

Vacuum suction massage, often used to stimulate lymphatic drainage and reduce fluid retention, works by sucking air out of a dome-shaped cup, simultaneously lifting the sub-cutaneous tissues as the unit is passed over the body, much in the way one would vacuum a carpet. Another variation on the same vacuum suction principle involves placing anything from four to eight vacuum cups of varying sizes, rather like pudding basins, on specific areas of the body. They are left in place for up to forty minutes while the tissues are sucked up, rolled and kneaded through the pumping action of the air. Suction force can be altered from gentle to very strong, depending on individial tolerance. This method is used to break down deposits of hard, lumpy fat on legs, hips, waist and bottom and redistribute them more smoothly and evenly. Treatments must be taken in close succession to one another, at the rate of no less than three a week. Widely-spaced single treatments do not achieve satisfactory results.

### Traditional steam treatments
*Sauna/Turkish bath/Steam cabinets*
One of the most popular myths among slimmers is that fat can be 'melted' away, merely by sufficient sweating. The truth, however, is that any weight-loss through perspiration is purely temporary and due entirely to the dehydrating effects of either dry heat as in a sauna, or steam heat used in Turkish baths and cabinets. Most, if not all weight lost through perspiration will automatically be regained once you take a drink after treatment. Taking a regular sauna or Turkish bath can help to boost sluggish circulation by dilating the blood vessels and increasing the flow of blood to the surface tissues. On its own, however, this is unlikely to have any effect on fluid retention or localised fat. Taking a heat treatment prior to a manual massage can help to relax the muscles and soften the skin, making the tissues more malleable and receptive to the masseur's hands.

## Hydrotherapy

Underwater massage has been used routinely for many years at spas and health clinics to stimulate the circulation and provide a tingly, toned-up sensation. Like heat treatments, however, it has little specific therapeutic value and is used principally as an adjunct to other methods. Hydro-massage may be applied via high-pressure jets of water to pummel the body from top to toe, or through a steady rhythmic force exerted underwater and aimed at specific areas, as in a jacuzzi. None of these has any effect on body shape, but by invigorating the system generally, can improve well-being if used just before or after a bout of vigorous exercise.

## Wax/Mud packs

The principle of applying warm or hot body packs is basically the same as other heat treatments – to induce perspiration. Because any natural substance such as mud will cool down rapidly, some salons increase the thermal action through a 'double wrap'. They apply a layer of wax or mud and then insulate the body further with a second layer of silver foil, plastic sheeting or blankets. In some cases, infra-red heat lamps are also used to 'bake' the body. Deeply relaxing, often to the point of radically reducing energy and inducing fatigue or sleep, the treatment can be useful in easing arthritis, alleviating muscular discomfort and joint pains. In terms of weight-loss, however, effects are the same as after a sauna or Turkish bath.

## High-tech reducing treatments

There is less mystique to these than the advertising buzz words and high-tech hype would have us believe. Electronic currents of various frequencies have been in use in clinics and beauty salons for a number of decades, and although the latest equipment may be more streamlined and fully automated, displaying as many dials and push buttons as a NASA control panel, the basic principles of treatment remain very much the same.

*Faradic current*

As used in passive exercise equipment (e.g. Slendertone), this is low frequency alternating current, omitted in rhythmic impulses which induces gentle, intermittent flexing and contraction of the muscles.

*Interferential current*

This is used increasingly in preference to the faradic current because it provides a smoother, more comfortable muscle contraction. Two medium frequency currents are applied to the body via two sets of electrodes, in such a way that the current flows cross each other within the muscle, causing a contraction. Passive exercise via this current tends to be less violent, more relaxing than with the faradic variety, which some people find produces a prickly and burning sensation. Widely used for sports injuries, lumbago, and muscular tension, many would-be slimmers get the erroneous impression that the current isn't working hard enough to exercise the muscles. In fact faradic and interferential currents are equally powerful and effective in creating muscular contractions.

Reports as to the figure-shaping potential of these methods vary greatly. Some salon clients do experience loss of inches (centimetres) due to muscular toning and tightening, especially around the thighs, particularly the inner area, and on the stomach, especially after childbirth. Others whose bodies are very flabby and unfit may see minimal improvement or even none at all. The general consensus of opinion amongst beauticians is that passive exercise machines fulfil a specific, if limited, function in toning up lazy muscles, prior to a regular, proper exercise programme.

**Machines aren't the lazy answer**

Electronic exercise machines are not an alternative to physical activity, only a useful adjunct under certain circumstances, as for example in the case of injury and post-natal body-shaping. In terms of time and cost, passive exercise can prove a non-viable proposition compared to taking exercise. A young, potentially fit person would have to undergo a daily one-hour treatment, the electronic unit turned up to an uncomfortably high level, for there to be any worthwhile effects. As it is, treatment should take place three times a week for 45 to 60 minutes at a time over a six-week period, during which time the clients are encouraged to switch over to some form of regular physical exercise.

*Galvanic current*

Also known as a direct current, because it flows in one direction, the galvanic current produces a constant muscle contraction and is therefore unsuitable for exercise equipment. However, it is used to introduce products and serums especially designed to counteract cellulite into the upper layers of the skin, through a process called Iontophoresis. A basic principle of physics is that opposite charges attract, so by applying a positively charged, water soluble serum to the skin and introducing a negatively charged current, the substance is then driven, via the transfer of positive ions, into the skin cells. There is a mild tingling sensation where pads attached to the negative and positive electrodes are strapped to the body. Anti-cellulite products used in Iontophoresis are usually plant-based, designed principally to improve circulation, dilate the blood vessels, decongest the tissues and counteract fluid retention.

The most advanced salon equipment used today to treat localised fat incorporates both faradic and galvanic electronic units. Therapists report that this two-pronged attack seems to achieve the fastest, most noticeable reduction and firming of body contours, although many emphasise the need to supplement electronic anti-cellulite treatment with a powerful massage to break up hardened fat even further, and improve elasticity and smoothness of the skin.

A number of combined passive exercise/Iontophoresis treatments have been extended even further to encompass the principles of heat treatment. The Inchaway M120 Ionithermie Treatment System incorporates an 'electro conducting' bodymask made of clay which hardens around areas of the body. It can also be applied to encase the entire body from breast to knees, retaining a high level of heat while the various electronically-charged pads underneath alternately induce muscular contraction, and encourage the penetration of anti-cellulite products. One of the selling points of this system is the guarantee of instant inch (centimetre) loss – anything from half to two inches (1.25 cm to 5 cm) on thighs or hips – after just one treatment. Testimonials abound, but the point is that this reduction, based on dehydration of the tissues, tends to be temporary and therefore, like any other course of reduction treatments, M120 must be supplemented with a regular exercise programme and weight control through diet. A course of eight to 12 sessions is generally recommended to achieve lasting benefits.

## Wrapping

Instant reduction in measurements of thighs, hips, waist, arms is also the chief appeal of a simple bandaging treatment (Kwikslim) where a herbal gel is applied to the skin and those parts of the body are then very tightly bandaged for about one and a half hours. Parts of the body may be reduced by up to two or three inches (5–7.5 cm) – measurements are taken before and after treatment. However, improvement works simply on the Cinderella principle, since reduction is strictly temporary, lasting sometimes no more than a few hours. To be fair, the manufacturers do not claim anything more long-lasting.

Effects are principally due to a shrinking of the tissues through dehydration, as fluid is squeezed out through pressure of the bandages. These must be applied extremely tightly to obtain results. Repeated treatments will maintain much of the intial loss, but only on the same temporary basis.

For anyone who wants, for just a few hours, to wear a dress or pair of trousers that have become prohibitively tight, this is probably a useful short-term strategy. Is it worth the money? It all depends on how desperate you are.

**Laser treatment**
Popular briefly a few years ago because of their supposed, and totally unsubstantiated, rejuvenating powers when applied to lines and wrinkles, lasers are now being used by some salons to treat localised fat and pitted 'orange peel' skin. Yesterday's trumped-up facial has been replaced by today's trumped-up body massage. What laser therapy amounts to is use of a fairly innocuous, low energy, infra-red laser-beam, instead of hand or machine, to stimulate circulation and decongest the tissues. Expensive, with at least a dozen sessions recommended before any improvement in body contours is seen, it is hard to detect any merit in this method. Reports of success are scant, even among therapists. This is not surprising, since lasers used for cosmetic purposes have all the power of the average battery torch and are therefore unlikely to have any significant effect on the dermal tissues.

**Mesotherapy**
A novel, if bizarre approach to spot reduction, which origi-nated in France, Mesotherapy is best known as an effective method of localised pain relief. It consists of a series of multiple

micro injections to introduce anti-cellulite extracts into the connective tissues. Treatment is given with either a multi-injector, an 8, 12 or 16-needle syringe more reminiscent of a medieval torture instrument than a modern implement of beauty, or a staple gun syringe. This latter is electronically programmed to give a series of intermittent injections of limited doses of serum into the tissues, as required. Areas commonly treated are the buttocks, hips, inner, outer, front and backs of thighs and the fleshy area inside and above the knee. Substances injected are largely plant-based and supposedly possess vasco-dilating and diuretic properties, aimed at improving circulation and reducing fluid retention.

Reports on efficacy vary, but some women claim to see a reduction in lumps and bulges after six to eight sessions, especially when treatment is accompanied by dietary restrictions and use of a mild diuretic. The injections can prove highly uncomfortable with lots of stinging and burning during treatment, followed by extensive unsightly bruising which may last for one or two weeks. Once the surplus fat has been reduced, therapists maintain that one or two booster sessions a year of Mesotherapy are needed to maintain overall improvement. This is a highly contentious claim, considering that individual lifestyle, diet, health and weight must inevitably influence localised fat distribution, as well as circulation and fluid retention.

# – 4 –
# *Home Treatments*

When it comes to skin-care or body-shaping, the average woman remains ever hopeful and credulous to a fault. The suggestion that a certain product can help cultivate a slimmer, tauter, younger-looking body is without doubt one of the most powerful of all marketing strategies. Like the promise that using this skin cream or that face mask may confer an everlasting youthful, wrinkle-free complexion, the lure of massage kits that purportedly melt away unsightly bulges is irresistible. Similarly attractive to many consumers is gadgetry which may intercept or reverse the inexorable downward pull of gravity on breasts or buttocks.

The sales figures attest to our willingness to give such things a try. We cherish the faint hope that one of these products may succeed in improving our figures. Deep down, the majority of clear thinkers may remain sceptical and dismissive, well aware that these products are almost certainly a waste of money. So what value, if any, is there in the proliferation of creams, oils, gadgets and gimmickry on the market for do-it-yourself would-be slimmers?

## Cellulite creams and kits
Like those best-selling, exotic, rejuvenating skin products that promise a reprieve from the ageing process, the rationale

behind all so called 'slimming' or 'recontouring' creams, gels, oils and lotions on the market is somewhat hard to take seriously. Body treatments, like anti-wrinkle creams, supposedly work by penetrating the living tissues. Yet the truth remains that there is as yet no scientific evidence to support the claims that cosmetic products, whether for face or body can penetrate any deeper than the epidermis.

*Superficial success*

On the other hand many oils, gels, masks and moisturisers on the market today do contain ingredients that can, in some cases, work very effectively. These products can tighten under-eye bags and puffy or slack skin, plump out fine lines and wrinkles, giving the temporary illusion of a smoother, tighter, younger skin. Even though thay may be superficial, the effects are often there to be seen, however temporarily.

*No change in shape*

But in contrast, when it comes to body contours, products that merely affect the skin surface can, by no conceivable stretch of the imagination, produce changes that might alter the quality or distribution of fatty tissue. What's more, products that superficially improve the skin of the body are hardly likely to have much effect on the fundamental contours. The breasts, for example, represent a completely inert weight made up entirely of fat and glandular tissue, veins and capillaries. Once this mass starts to sag due to pregnancy, breast-feeding, weight-gain or the combined forces of gravity and time, the skin gradually becomes over stretched and distends. No amount of massage or application of treatment products can halt, prevent or even slow down the process.

The same goes for stomach tissues. Once the abdominal tissues have lost their elasticity through weight-gain, pregnancy, or both, then no amount of surface beauty treatments will make them regain their former suppleness and smoothness. This is illustrated by the fact that even after fat has been lost through dieting, and exercise has restored the tummy muscles to their former tone and strength, loose surplus flesh may linger to give an impression of slack, sagging contours. Women whose skin is still taut and unmarked *during* pregnancy may, however, minimise their chances of developing stretch marks by applying a rich skin cream or body oil to stomach, breast and thigh tissues. This will keep them soft and supple, and prevent the dehydration and loss of elasticity that can result from pregnancy.

*Stimulating treatment for cellulite*

The main selling point behind a growing number of bath additives, creams, gels and oils is their ability to counteract or bannish cellulite – localised flab or lumpy, bumpy, puckered 'orange peel' skin (of which more in Chapter 3) on thighs, hips and bottoms. According to manufacturers, the rationale for 'the anti-cellulite action' of such products is the effect of diverse plant extracts such as ivy, seaweed, gingseng, etc. These, they say, stimulate blood circulation, lymph drainage and cellular activity of the skin's connective tissue. Claims that these ingredients can enhance the living tissues remain unsubstantiated, and due to increasingly stricter legislation on advertising, have become comparatively modest.

Those in whom hope springs eternal would do well, however, to remember that there is no proof whatever that any substance massaged into the skin's surface can 'dissolve' or 'unclog' fat cells, release 'trapped toxins', 'eliminate excess fluid', to use some of the current jargon of the beauty trade. The hype has been toned down considerably however, and all that the most reputable manufacturers now suggest is that regular use of their products may improve the surface appearance of such trouble spots as dimple thighs.

The French company Vichy report that in a survey of 200 women replying to a questionnaire published in two health magazines, 87 per cent found that regular use of the hip and thigh cream left their skin more supple and soft, reducing the orange peel effect. There are, however, no conclusive reports of any significant improvement in body shape, or reduction in measurement of hips or thighs.

As a toning, softening treatment therefore, the anti-cellulite products do seem to have some value – provided they are used properly. This seems to be where the main problem lies. Any type of do-it-yourself home regime, be it exercise or massage, must be carried out regularly in order to produce any significant result. But most people with busy lives and little time to spend on themselves will give up after a few desultory attempts at self-massage because of the time, effort and discipline required.

The body contouring kits all carry instructions for regular once or twice daily use over a period of ten to 21 days. The creams should be massaged into the affected areas after bath or shower, while the skin is still warm and thus capable of absorbing the product more effectively. Placing a lot of faith in the creams themselves, the manufacturers stress that the results may be obtained by simply rubbing the product in by hand, although some firms sell rubber hand massage units or gloves. These feature elevated ribs or nodules to provide a more intensive and vigorous professional-style massage.

*Massage kits*
Provided you have sufficient dedication and discipline, as well as a strong pair of hands, massage to soften and smooth minor lumpiness and even out pitted or dimpled skin on the thighs and pep up circulation, is a cheap and effective method of self-help. Massage *must* be regular – preferably a five to ten-minute session every day – if it is to produce any results in stimulating

the circulation and softening hardened, lumpy tissues. Do-it-yourself massage mimmicks that practised by professional masseurs. Concentrate on strong, firm, upward strokes with the pads of fingers, pinching, kneading and twisting. Use both the hands as if working on a lump of dough. Movements should be deep and firm, but not so vigorous that you bruise the flesh or experience pain.

Using an anti-cellulite cream or oil helps the fingers slide more easily over the tissues and allows for a much deeper, probing massage. Using a rubber massage glove, such as those made by Helancyl or Biotherm, takes some of the finger-aching slog out of the whole exercise.

*Getting to grips with the body*

Areas that are easier to get to grips with in order to carry out a thorough massage are the front and sides of the thighs, hips and the flesh round and above the knees. Consequently, these areas tend to firm up well in response to regular massage. More difficult, because slightly out of reach, are backs of thighs and buttocks, so it makes more sense to use a massage glove on these areas. Beware of scrubbing or digging too zealously, as this can damage the skin and may even cause stretch marks by breaking the delicate surface skin tissues.

*The rough stuff*

Other massage aids available in beauty salons or department stores include loofahs, or mitts, made of rough, scratchy material such as hemp or synthetic materials. These look and feel rather like scouring pads adapted for use on human flesh. Although they have no reducing effects whatsoever on body contours, used vigorously with soap in the bath or shower in a brisk, circular motion, they provide a stimulating friction massage. This refines and softens the skin and temporarily increases the flow of blood to the surface. The warm, tingling sensation also imparts a feeling of fitness and well-being which is largely psychological, but nevertheless a valuable adjunct to the whole business of body-care and reshaping.

### Gadgetry: Passive exercise

The appeal of passive exercise equipment – just strap on a couple of pads to the areas that need tightening and lie back while the machine does all the work – isn't hard to understand. In theory, machines like Slendertone are a godsend to the lazy and weak-willed, who nevertheless wish to retain the trim, taut body of someone who works out regularly. But how well do these machines shape up the body, if at all?

To begin with, this passive method will only have a chance of working for you if you are generally slim all over, with perhaps one or two stubborn problem areas that never seem to respond to dieting or simple exercise. For example, areas such as the tummy, waistline, inner thighs, tops of thighs and buttocks, which can all prove notoriously difficult to trim down or tone up. Some women and men do report excellent improvements through passive exercise, but then others remain disappointed in spite of hours spent strapped up and plugged in, muscles twitching and jumping, in response to electronic stimuli.

*Hitting the spot*

Experts claim that a lot of it is trial and error, since much depends on finding the correct areas on which to strap the pads. It may take an expert therapist with years of training in operating such equipment to locate the exact spot on which to attach the pads. Since no two bodies are identical, this will inevitably vary from individual to individual, depending on physical type, muscle strength and weaknesses, and a particular reshaping need of that person.

Having successfully located the target zone, problem

number two is zeroing in on it correctly at each treatment. Since this is a challenge to even the most experienced therapist, the likelihood of an untrained man or woman, a novice to the whole science of muscle groups, getting the best out of the equipment is obviously much less. After all, during all forms of exercise, from swimming and running to calisthenics, the body moves in a natural, integrated fashion. You do not instruct isolated muscle groups as to how they must move, unless of course you are working-out in a gym or using weights, i.e., body-building. Muscle groups all work spontaneously, in a co-ordinated way. The problem with passive electronic exercise is that it is selective – you choose which bits of your body you want to exercise. What's more it is self-selected, so failure to derive benefit may be due more to lack of expertise than mechanical failure.

Equipment such as the Slendertone unit for home use is not cheap, so in order to find out whether this method could be the answer to those flabby thighs or sagging tummy muscles try a few sessions at a reputable beauty salon or borrow a unit from a friend. It is important to remember that machines such as Slendertone have no effect on areas of excess fat, nor will the machine transform arms, thighs, waist, tummy or buttocks that are chronically outsize.

*Benefits of exercise machines*

Where passive exercise can help is in strengthening and tightening muscles that have become slack through lack of use. Electronic gadgetry also offers an alternative to older people or those with health problems such as high blood pressure, which might prevent them from exercising. For example, someone suffering from a chronic back problem which obviously precludes strenuous tummy exercises, might find passive exercise an ideal method of strengthening muscles and reducing a flabby stomach. The system is completely safe, and there is also no danger of over-exercising the muscles and building the sort of ugly bulk associated with weight-lifters.

Ideally, the passive method should be augmented by proper exercise. Electronic stimulation can also strengthen and prime untoned lazy muscles for a future exercise programme, especially after injury, illness, pregnancy or a prolonged bout of inactivity. Geared to exercise specific isolated muscle groups, it is, therefore, by definition, no substitute for a balanced exercise programme. It could, however, prove a valuable adjunct for someone with stubborn, localised problems.

*How it works*

The principle behind electro-muscular stimulation, which is extensively used in hospital for sports injury and rehabilitation, is simple to understand. When voluntarily contracting a muscle during any form of exercise the brain transmits a signal along a nerve to the motor point of that muscle. Similar to a weak electric current, this message 'tells' the muscle to contract. In the case of passive exercise, electrodes in the form of conductive rubber pads are strapped onto the body, in contact with the motor points of specific muscles. A weak electronic current (faradic current) is then transmitted via the pads, stimulating the motor points and thereby causing the muscles to contract.

This regular rhythm of alternating contractions and relaxation should be comfortable and soothing. Eight or more pads can be applied at a time, depending on individual needs, and the strength of contractions can be altered by controlling a dial on the unit. In a 35-minute session, faradic equipment can give over 1,000 separate contractions to those muscles being treated. Manufacturers of equipment such as Slendertone stress that in order to obtain noticeable results, treatment should take place every day, if possible, for at least 35 minutes at a time. They emphasise, however, that if figure problems are partly due to excess fat, then treatment should be backed up by some form of weight-reducing diet.

*Boredom is the drawback*
Machines such as Slendertone do seem to work for many people, usually in cases where a fairly active person of normal weight simply wants to tighten areas such as the upper and inner thigh or the stomach and waist, especially after childbirth or a long period of inactivity. The most obvious drawback is boredom. People with even a limited amount of physical energy to spare tend to feel they are not doing anything vigorous or positive to improve the body, hence this can be a very unsatisfactory method of reshaping. Few people have patience, let alone the spare time, to lie or sit for over half an hour each day strapped up in rubber pads and hooked into an exercise machine. Thus the drop-out rate among home users tends to be high.

Because results are far from instant, with improvements visible only after a reasonable length of time, say two to three weeks of daily use, many passive exercisers also tend to give up or slow down treatment through lack of immediate motivation or encouragement, coupled with a sense that unlike active exercise, one cannot push oneself more arduously along the road to fitness.

## Weight-loss garments
Made of synthetic fabric, various makes of 'sweatsuits' have been available on the market for years. Some are designed to be worn while exercising to increase perspiration and, more sensibly, to keep the muscles warm and so protect against injury, especially when training in a cold environment. Although worn by a large number of students and pro-

fessional dancers during classes and rehearsals, often in the vain hope that extra sweating may induce weight-loss, all that happens when the body perspires more readily and excessively is a very temporary and minor drop in weight, due to fluid loss. Weight rises again as soon as the lost fluid is replaced after exercising. Sweat 'knickers' or plastic boiler suits, whether worn during exercise or while doing household chores, are therefore of no value in shaping the body or losing weight.

*Getting in a sweat*
Although they can also prove extremely irritating and uncomfortable when worn for keep-fit sessions, especially in hot weather, insulating the body and cultivating your own tropical 'micro climate' while you work-out can help psychologically. It makes you feel you are getting the most out of your exercise regime! After all, sweating profusely during a class or workout is usually the acid test of whether you are doing it to the best of your abilities, which is rather unfair on someone who simply does not sweat readily or profusely when exercising. Wearing sweat garments while just sitting down and watching TV for example, is, however, a complete waste of time and will have no effect on the body whatsoever.

# – 5 –
# *Exercise*

There can be little argument about the body-shaping benefits of exercise. Together with eating a well-balanced diet, exercising regularly is without any doubt the soundest possible investment you could make in maintaining physical fitness and tone. Not that exercise will transform you if you are overweight – there is no chance that it will. But what it will almost certainly do is strengthen and firm up body contours, tighten and tone flabby or slack muscles and discourage you from putting on weight in the first place.

Backed up by an effective weight-reducing diet, certain forms of exercise can help encourage faster weight-loss by stimulating a more rapid burn up of Calories (kilojoules). They can also produce rapid and visible results through shaping up, tightening and adding definition to certain parts of the body. In the case of minor weight problems – say up to no more than half a stone (3 kg) of excess weight – regular exercise may sometimes be sufficient to eliminate those extra pounds (kilogrammes), provided your Calorie (kilojoule) intake is not increased to 'make up' for any extra physical exertion!

**Does exercise help you lose weight?**
The number of fitness enthusiasts who can testify to the

figure-shaping and reducing benefits of exercise are today legion. Yet controversy still abounds regarding the merits of exercise in reducing or slimming the body. The profuse sweating that results from physical exertion may cause a temporary weight-reduction through fluid loss, but the weight is regained when that fluid is replaced. Most dietitians and doctors argue, therefore, that exercise has little value in any slimming programme because the amount of physical exertion needed to burn up even a few extra Calories (kilojoules), rather than sweat away some excess fluid, is excessively high.

Up to a point this is of course perfectly true: in order to burn 100 Calories (420 kilojoules) you would have to run one mile in six minutes and to lose one pound (½ kilogramme) through exercise you would have to burn 3,500 Calories (14.7 megajoules). It is a salutary thought that every pound (kilogramme) of excess fat equals 3,500 Calories (14.7 megajoules) that you haven't burned. Being 7 lbs (3 kg) overweight, therefore, represents 24,500 unused Calories (102.9 megajoules) – or taken over one year, about 70 Calories (29.4 kilojoules) a day that are transformed straight into fat. If you are 10 lbs (3.8 kg) overweight you can reckon that around 100 Calories (420 kilojoules) a day are going to fat.

However, those people who merely want to lose perhaps three or four extra pounds (one or two kilogrammes), gained over a period of winter bingeing or inactivity, could lose about one pound (½ kilogramme) every two weeks by burning 200–250 Calories (840–1,050 kilojoules) daily through exercise. In theory at any rate, 14 weeks of regular daily exercise without any dietary restrictions could be all you need to drop 7 lbs (3 kg) in weight, provided you are not over 150 lb (66 kg) in the first place. Doctor Kenneth Cooper of the Aerobics Centre, Dallas, Texas, has worked out a rough guide to how much exercise and time this might take.

| Activity | Calories burnt per hour | Megajoules burnt per hour | Time needed to burn 250 Calories (1.05 megajoules) |
|---|---|---|---|
| Skating (Moderate) | 354 | 1.5 | 42 minutes |
| Walking (4–5 mph) | 400 | 1.7 | 37 " |
| Tennis (Moderate) | 425 | 1.8 | 35 " |
| Swimming (Crawl, 45 yd/min) | 530 | 2.2 | 28 " |
| Downhill Skiing | 585 | 2.4 | 26 " |
| Handball, Squash | 600 | 2.5 | 25 " |
| Tennis (Vigorous) | 600 | 2.5 | 25 " |
| Jogging (5.5 mph) | 650 | 2.7 | 23 " |
| Cycling (13 mph) | 850 | 3.8 | 18 " |

**Raising metabolic rate**

Researchers into the effects of exercise on body metabolism claim that regular periods of aerobic exercise, for example, jogging, swimming, cycling, carried out uninterruptedly for ten to 20 minutes at a time, may help to crank up the body's metabolism (the rate at which calories (kilojoules) are burnt up as a source of energy). Some exercise physiologists believe that Calories (kilojoules) continue to be burnt up at a faster rate, not only during physical activity, but also for a considerable period afterwards. Effects of a raised metabolic rate depend on how long and vigorously you work-out, and at which type of exercise.

A number of theories, none yet fully proven, have been put forward for this raised metabolic rate. One claim is that, because it works-out major muscle groups, aerobic exercise causes loss of fat and a proportional increase of lean tissue, which is believed to be more metabolically active at all times in a person who exercises regularly. The reason for this, according to some exercise physiologists, is that aerobic exercise promotes the activity of what has been called 'red' or 'fast twitch' muscle fibre, which is the type most needed for activities requiring endurance and stamina. Long distance runners, for instance, have a higher percentage of red muscle fibre than sprinters, for example.

The chief fuel used by working muscles is glycogen, a derivative of glucose which is stored in the muscles and the liver. In addition, red muscle fibre uses up quantities of the body's fat stores to make up an extra source of energy. Whereas glycogen stores are topped up almost instantly to provide the body with ready energy, fat is not necessarily replaced so readily.

## Why sitting makes you fat

It has been argued that people with sedentary lives often become fat, not because they eat large quantities of food, but because red muscle degenerates through lack of use, lowering the body's metabolism. Another hypothesis is that if you have less red muscle you will put on weight more easily, even when eating fairly modest amounts, and will be less able to burn off fat through exercise.

The corollary to this argument is of course very beguiling – it is claimed that people who exercise regularly can eat more and gain no extra fat, while inactive people who don't eat more have a weight problem. It is an argument that dietitians and metabolic researchers dismiss as highly contentious. In fact, the opposite seems to apply. If you talk to many dedicated exercise enthusiasts who train regularly, although perhaps not at marathon level, the general consensus seems to be that they eat less, not more.

## Exercise beats hunger

Vigorous exercise seems more often to suppress than to stimulate appetite, and there appears to be a good biochemical explanation for this. When your blood sugar level drops, you feel hungry. Regular exercise elevates and stabilises blood sugar as the muscles use up proportionately more fat than sugar as fuel, controlling hunger as well as depleting stored fat. People who exercise regularly tend to have more energy because of elevated and stable glycogen levels. They may, therefore, become generally more physically active and thus liable to burn off Calories (kilojoules) at a faster rate than someone with a sedentary lifestyle. Obviously, the more you can cut down on Calorie (kilojoule) intake and step up Calorie (kilojoule) combustion through exercise, the better the combined slimming effects of diet control and exercise.

Whichever way you look at it, the benefits of exercise are undeniable – except of course if you are chronically lazy, unfit and determined to remain so.

**Exercise for all**

It is now generally acknowledged that exercise need not be all masochistic slog to do you good. You don't have to achieve the Jane Fonda 'burn' to do yourself good. You could become fitter doing some much gentler form of exercise. Keeping fit these days has lost its 'fanatic' tag. According to Doctor Kenneth Cooper, all you need to do is exercise six times a week for 12 to 20 minutes at between 70 and 85 per cent of your normal maximum heart rate to obtain the aerobic 'training effect' necessary to boost metabolism, as well as provide the heart and lungs with an effective work-out. This training effect can be obtained for example just by:

Running one mile (1.5 km) in less than eight minutes/stationary running for 12½ minutes.

Swimming 600 yards (545 m) in less than 15 minutes.

Cycling five miles (8 km) in less than 20 minutes.

Running on the spot for 12½ minutes.

Walking two miles (3 km) in 24 to 30 minutes, or three miles (5 km) in 36 to 43 minutes.

Put that way, exercise surely becomes the art of the possible. Don't let the sport ethic daunt you. Never mind that five mile (8 km) dawn jog or marathon endurance level. We can *all*, even if relatively busy, lazy or initially unfit, take up some form of exercise and achieve a relative level of fitness which will confer tremendous benefits. And it is worth remembering that, while there is still no hard scientific evidence that exercise can make you live longer and avoid getting heart disease, evidence for slimming and shaping potential is clearly visible. Just take up a regular exercise programme for a month or so and then look at your body. Even if you do not lose weight, the chances are that any regular activity, even if non-aerobic, will improve the shape and tone of the body, reducing inches, tightening contours and removing flab. These are all effects that are sometimes hard to achieve through dieting alone.

The question therefore, for everyone who is truly committed to achieving a slim, firm, well-proportioned body is not, Why exercise? but, What exercise? No activity, be it daily dozen, aerobic burn-up, or gym training should be die-hard and doctrinaire. Enjoyment is one of the prime criteria in choosing how to keep fit. Keeping sight of the pleasure principle while exercising is more likely to turn you into a passionate enthusiast than a duty-bound stalwart.

### Choosing your type of exercise

Nor is there any perfect one-for-all system as far as exercise goes. Temperament, health, lifestyle, age, body type, environment, must all to a degree dictate our choice of exercise. Much is a matter of trial and error. If you already walk a lot, jogging may appeal as a natural extension, but a couple of trial runs could be enough to spell boredom. If you are gregarious, confident and love pop music, keep fit classes could well fit the bill, while the athletically inclined may be instinctively drawn to gym, swimming-pool or tennis-court.

Knowing what suits you is half the battle. The other half is being able to identify which exercise method does what for you, and how much time and effort you need to invest in order to get the most out of it. A very slim man or woman of normal weight may embark on an intensive programme of weight-lifting in the gym to build muscles, but this, of course, will have little effect on metabolism. A woman with heavy thighs and large bottom may lose weight jogging regularly but find that her basic pear-shape remains unaltered. Different types of exercise, as explained in the following pages, tend to have different effects on the body and specific activities will inevitably focus on individual areas of the body.

## All-round exercise

The most comprehensive and well-balanced exercise regime is one that includes the best elements of each type of exercise. You do not concentrate on one aspect of fitness to the complete exclusion of others. You can exercise to improve stamina, suppleness, posture and alignment, coordination, bodily strength – or all of these.

Being as flexible as a rubber doll does not mean that you necessarily have the stamina to run three miles, while someone with rotten posture can still run a marathon, though their body may look unaligned and bulky in repose. Pumping iron can provoke a muscular metamorphosis and give you dramatically different body proportions, while doing little to improve flexibility and strength. The gentler forms of exercise such as yoga, medau, T'ai Chi, can alter body shape only minimally, yet improve the intrinsic posture and alignment of the entire body, giving an impression of slimness, poise, added height where once the body was slouched, tense, flabby and weak.

## Check your bad points

The most common pitfall to avoid is 'exercising in' any postural faults or weaknesses such as hunched shoulders, sagging tummy, sway-back. Before embarking on any form of regular exercise check and try to become aware of any unconscious bad habits you might have, in particular while standing and walking. Try to prevent these distorting your body while you run, walk, cycle, do fitness classes or weight-training.

Unlike skilled sports and team games which are great for those who have the time and aptitude for them, general exercise can be enjoyed by virtually everybody of any age, provided they are in reasonably good health. If in doubt, you must obtain your doctor's approval before beginning regular exercise, especially if you are over thirty-five or forty and have not exercised regularly for years, or have suffered a serious injury or illness.

### Doing what comes naturally

On the whole, it is best to stick to an activity that you feel happy doing and which suits the needs of your body as well as your personality. It should also be one you can manage to carry out reasonably well. Clearly, attempting to take up tennis in the mid thirties or forties if you are unfit, as well as a stranger to the tennis court, is as unwise as it is unrealistic. Your chances of deriving either pleasure or fitness from it are few.

Ideally, any good, all-round exercise should combine plenty of stretching movements to keep the muscles and limbs supple; all-out exertion to give the heart and lungs a full work-out and raise the level of circulation and metabolism; and rhythmic muscle contractions to strengthen all the main muscle groups. If you lead a stressful and rather competitive life, it is best to steer clear of aggressive games like squash, where the emphasis is on winning, as you could unconsciously add to your stress levels by trying to beat your opponent – or worse, by losing the game!

Dancing, cycling, running, fast walking, swimming and gym exercises are all good non-competitive, all-round activities that allow you to set your own pace. They should suit just about everyone who wants to exercise in order to keep fit and trim, rather than to win or set new goals.

**Before you start**
A thorough five-minute warm-up before starting any form of exercise is an essential part of minimising the risk of injury to joints, muscles or ligaments. Exercising on a full stomach interferes with the digestion and can cause nausea and cramp, so wait for two hours after you have eaten. On the other hand, exercising when you are hungry has the almost magic effect of instantaneously diminishing or removing appetite altogether. This operates during and for a while after physical activity. You can learn to set your cue for exercise when you might otherwise be sitting down to a fattening snack.

To do any good at all, exercise must be regular. Better five or ten minutes a day than an occasional exhausting marathon session once a week. Doing 20 to 30 minutes every other day is ideal: working out for two hours or more on Sundays only isn't, and may even prove physically harmful. Setting aside a regular time of day or evening and sticking to it, instead of embarking on sporadic bursts of activity every now and then, with long periods of inactivity in between, will help you incorporate physical exercise into your daily life. This will encourage you to build up stamina and strength, and it will produce the fastest, most visible changes in body shape.

―― *WHICH EXERCISE? A CHOICE OF THE ACTION* ――

**Aerobic Exercise**
Any activity which increases the amount of oxygen intake until you begin to huff and puff and break out in a sweat is aerobic. The activity shouldn't make you completely breath-

less, and ideally you could carry on a slightly 'breathy' conversation while exercising. Most obvious examples are jogging, running, fast walking, cycling, swimming, dancing.

To achieve what Doctor Kenneth Cooper calls the necessary 'training effect', especially important for giving heart and lungs a proper work-out, the activity must be kept up continuously for more than 12 minutes. It must be carried out vigorously enough to raise and sustain the heart rate to 120 or more beats per minute. If exercising doesn't raise the heart rate to this level, then it should be carried out for longer periods.

*Time involved* – Frequent. Three, four or preferably daily sessions per week are the key to building up cardiovascular strength and improving endurance levels, though each session need last no longer than 20 to 30 minutes. Short, intensive bouts at any time of day or evening are obviously appealing to anyone with a busy schedule.

*Weight-loss/body-shaping benefits* – Regular aerobic exercise builds cardiovascular fitness superbly. This means a stronger heart and lungs and improved circulation. It also encourages larger, more flexible blood vessels and more efficient metabolism. Many people find the so-called training effect causes gradual weight-loss due to raised metabolism. Overall stamina as well as body strength develops steadily as you train.

A word about the much vaunted 'burn'. Unless you are extremely fit – don't go for it. The burning sensation is caused by accumulation of lactic acid, a chemical by-product of vigorous exercise, in muscle. It will not cause fat to 'melt away'. It merely encourages muscle fatigue and increases the risk of injury. By burning extra Calories (kilojoules) you may well replace a certain amount of body fat with lean muscle tissue, firming and trimming the body over a longer period. But because, pound for pound, (kilogramme for kilogramme) muscle weighs more than fat, you may start to look slimmer while weighing the same or even more.

Swimming gives every muscle group in the body a full, smooth, coordinated work-out, without risk of strain or injury. It also develops elongated streamlined contours. Cycling strengthens thighs and tummy and tightens inner thighs. Fast walking tightens leg contours, while running firms the thighs and whittles hips. But in general, aerobic exercise has more of an effect on cardiovascular fitness and overall metabolism than on actual contours.

*Is it right for you?* It is if you like solitary activities, are non-competitive and want a cheap, uncomplicated, get-up-and-go fitness plan that you can build into your working day – e.g. cycling or walking to work, jogging in the lunch-hour, swimming in the early evening after work. Swimming is the single most ideal, all-round exercise for anyone who is unfit or suffers from a back injury.

*Drawbacks* – Jogging, walking, cycling, swimming can get monotonous and you may miss the body-shaping element. You may become obsessed by setting ever higher personal goals, with a risk of injury and exhaustion. You can avoid both by alternating aerobic with other forms of exercise or combining various permutations of aerobic activity, e.g. swimming, cycling and running, or walking, swimming and dancing.

### Dance

By its very nature, most dancing is an aerobic activity, provided you keep going non-stop for at least 12 minutes during any one class. However, the currently popular aerobic dance systems incorporate continuous skipping, bouncing, running on the spot and kicking, along with stretching, flexing, strengthening exercises that are part of standard keep fit or jazz dance classes. The new 'low impact aerobics' system is less frenetic and gruelling and involves less risk of damage to the joints, because one foot or both feet are always kept on the floor while the rest of the body is in motion. Ballet, tap, modern jazz have all become popular recently as fun, stimulating exercise for non-professionals.

*Time involved* – Most dance classes are one to one-and-a-half hours, and you need to go twice or more times a week to gain full benefits and overcome initial stiffness, as well as learning difficulties. However, you can study and practise at home once you have learnt the basics, using a well-written, clearly illustrated book for guidance.

*Weight-loss/body-shaping benefits* – Cardiovascular endurance, improved flexibility of the joints, suppleness and strengthening and lengthening of the muscles, especially of the lower body. Dance grabs concentration and imagination, involves the challenge of learning new skills and opens up the opportunities of self-expression and creativity. It turns your attention away from everyday problems. It is therefore a terrific antidote to stress, tension, depression and anxiety. Dance can also prove a great self-confidence booster.

Body-shaping potential is good, provided you work out at least three times a week in class or at home, but don't expect to see significant results for the first month or two – a dancer's body must be tuned slowly and gently. Weight-loss may occur as a spin off from increased metabolism which burns off fat, but you may develop extra muscle tissue which tends to weigh more.

Ballet, jazz, aerobic dance and 'California stretch', e.g. the Jane Fonda Work-out, all tend to streamline the thighs, firm and lift the buttocks, tighten the stomach, firm the hips and waist, and eliminate any 'spare tyre'. The Lotte Berk system is tough and renowned for shaping legs, tightening and firming the bottom, thighs and hips. There is sometimes a danger of over-straining or doing the exercises incorrectly. This may not only cause joint or muscle injury, but cultivate unattractive bunched or bulky leg muscles.

Try to watch a class before joining in yourself. Check that

the teacher spends enough time correcting and demonstrating slowly and clearly and does not push unfit beginners too far or too fast.

*Is it for you?* – It is if you are basically unathletic but energetic, love music, perhaps studied dance as a child, are physically fairly well co-ordinated, and have an element of the extrovert about you. You should also have time and enough self-discipline to work at home if you can't always get to class.

*Drawbacks* – The time, cost of classes, eventual monotony if you only go to the same teacher. There are also the dangers of bad teachers, overcrowded classes and risk of muscular soreness and injury.

### Calisthenics

These are simple but vigorous exercises such as sit ups, side bends, toe touching, arm swings, etc. They flex the joints, tone and stretch the muscles, and are often incorporated into aerobics, dance or keep fit classes. Calisthenics may also be used to warm up before aerobics or other sports activities.

*Time involved* – A good beneficial work-out should last 15 to 30 minutes and be done at least three times a week. Do calisthenics at home, in a keep fit or aerobic dance class, gym or health club, or alone with the help of one of the many books on the market.

*Weight loss/body-shaping benefits* – Provided you build up to a very fast, uninterrupted work-out for at least 12 to 15 minutes, and minimise the rest period between exercises, the system will increase cardiovascular fitness and stamina while stretching and strengthening joints and muscles. If you carry out a really vigorous and fast 12 to 15 minute routine, you can burn around 120 Calories (5.04 megajoules) at a time (the same guide applies to a dance class).

Body shaping potential is excellent, especially if you tailor the exercises to focus on specific problem areas such as waist, thighs, tummy, hips, etc. Improved muscle tone will eventually make you look slimmer, but don't expect rapid results. You can use light weights strapped onto ankles and wrists to achieve a tougher work-out.

*Is it for you?* – It is if you like an adaptable programme, yet one that's relatively uncomplicated and simple to learn. Excellent for anyone who wants to exercise at home, even in the garden, a hotel room, wherever there is enough room to move arms and legs freely. Disco or beat music encourages rhythmic and co-ordinated movements and keeps spirits up.

*Drawbacks* – These are very few. This is probably the most universally popular system of exercise for the fit and active, as well as for the relatively unfit. If you exercise at home with just a book for guidance there is a slight danger of doing the exercises incorrectly and therefore deriving fewer benefits. Home work-outs can also prove notoriously boring, and you need steely self-discipline to do them regularly, even if you work-out with the aid of a video such as the *Jane Fonda Work-out tape*.

### Gym training (free weights)

This involves either using barbells while doing calisthenics and/or using your body to move machinery against the resistance of weights. The weights can be altered to give greater or lesser resistance and therefore a tougher or easier work-out. There are machines designed to exercise nearly every part of the body and you are given a 'circuit' or programme to suit your individual ability and changing needs.

*Time involved* – About 20 to 30 minutes, three times a week. Longer work-outs are counter-productive because of muscle fatigue. You will need to join a gym or health club – the cost varies according to location and other amenities offered. If using free weights only (e.g. dumb-bells) you can do a fairly comprehensive work-out at home. Home exercise equipment such as Bullworkers or multi-action all-in-one gym machines work well in theory because you can adapt them to exercise different parts of the body, but in practice the home gym work-out is a boring slog, with a notoriously high drop out rate.

*Weight-loss/body shaping benefits* – Weight training will primarily strengthen the muscles, improving flexibility, though on conventional equipment you will derive little in the way of all-round stamina or cardiovascular fitness. Body shaping potential is absolutely superb and can be extremely fast. Rapid, visible reshaping is what weight training is all about. Regular work-outs will slim and shape the legs, tighten flabby thighs, flatten and lift the buttocks, flatten tummy, trim the waist, build the upper arms and chest, improve bust contours, generally define the muscles and streamline the contours. This is a great way to lose inches, though weight-loss may be minimal – indeed, by developing the muscles you may actually end up weighing more. To burn up extra Calories (kilojoules), use moderate weights and work up to as many repetitions as possible. Contrary to popular misconception, women do *not* build large bulky muscles in the Charles Atlas mould, because of the lack of necessary male hormones.

*Is it for you?* – It is if you want visible body contouring results fast, and don't mind a bit of monotony and slog to get there. Also if you like to work under guidance, in the company of others in a clubby atmosphere and don't mind paying a membership or entry fee to enjoy gym facilities.

*Drawbacks* – Principally the boredom of doing a repetitive, simple work-out, and risk of injury if you don't use the machines properly. There should always be an instructor to keep an eye on you, especially when you are just beginning this system of training. Definitely not recommended for anyone with a weak or injured back, or joint problems. Popular gym centres can become crowded, especially early in the morning, during lunch-time and after work: there is sometimes a queue to use machines, which means you cool down when you don't want to.

### Omnikinetic resistance (Hydrafitness)

A recent development in resistance training using equipment (i.e. Hydrafitness machinery), whose resistance is controlled by hydraulic cylinders, not metal weights. Instead of 'pumping iron' you are 'pushing liquid'. This offers a variety of advantages over ordinary gym equipment. Body movement is smooth and co-ordinated, because the user generates his or her own force. The equipment continuously accommodates that strength, and varies with it, from the weakest to the strongest point in any range of motion.

Two sets of complementary muscle groups can be exercised simultaneously, giving a 'concentric' work-out in which you carry out two different sorts of exercise at the same time. For example, you pull to lift your arm up and then have to push to bring it down again, instead of allowing the limb to be forced back to the starting position. The results include a more intensive and thorough work-out of each muscle group, no risk of injury or muscle soreness and stiffness following exercise.

*Time involved* – Three or four 28-minute sessions per week.

*Weight-loss/body shaping benefits* – Unlike weight training using conventional machinery, Hydrafitness requires stamina rather than strength, takes less time than ordinary weight training and provides first-class aerobic exercise. An average work-out takes only about 28 minutes and is claimed to burn up 400 Calories (1.68 megajoules) – approximately equal to an hour's jogging. Weight-loss, as well as speedy body slimming and shaping, is reported by many regular users of Hydrafitness. This type of equipment can be used to good effect even by the very unfit or elderly and anyone recovering from an injury. The system is more likely to build a streamlined, swimmer's body than a muscley, athletic one.

*Is it right for you?* – This is the ideal method of exercise for anybody who has minimum time to devote to exercise, yet wants a good aerobic and muscle strengthening work-out. Over a period of time, however, it can become as monotonous and boring as all other forms of weight training, since the range of exercises are, by their very nature rather limited. All in all, this offers many worthwhile improvements on old-style weight training. It should appeal to men and women who are looking for a short, safe, uncomplicated and painless exercise routine that reshapes and trims the body. It has the additional bonus of a cardiovascular work-out and increased Calorie (kilojoule) burn-up.

*Drawbacks* – There are none, except that Hydrafitness is not yet widely installed in fitness and gym centres in some countries.

## Pilates

Much favoured by dancers, actors, singers, the system was devised to strengthen and stretch every part of the body without strain or risk of injury. A variety of stretching and limbering exercises based on ballet and yoga are carried out on machines fitted with tension springs. These springs provide varying degrees of resistance and therefore give muscles an optimum work-out. Emphasis is on performing fluid, smoothly co-ordinated movements, backed up with rhythmic and relaxed breathing patterns.

*Time involved* – Sessions are anything from one to two hours, depending on how basic and simple, or extended and elaborate, your personal 'routine'. Two or three sessions a week are recommended and after a course of ten you should begin to see and feel results.

*Weight-loss/body shaping benefits* – Benefits are in relaxation, body control and co-ordination, improvement of injuries, weaknesses and back problems. All exercises are performed lying down, so the system is ideal for anyone with back problems or women who are pregnant or very unfit. There is no risk of injury – even non beginners receive one-to-one instruction and supervision. Exercises encourage sleekness rather than bulk, cultivating a dancer's rather than an athlete's body. Emphasis is on strengthening the upper and lower abdominal muscles, thereby flattening the tummy, narrowing the waistline, tightening the inner and outer thighs, pulling up and firming the buttocks.

*Is it right for you?* – It is if you are prepared to work hard and concentrate. Don't expect to cheat by doing the exercises incorrectly. Pilates requires dedication and commitment. You need the ability to tune in to your own breathing and identify isolated areas of the body, including specific muscle groups, in order to get them all working correctly.

*Drawbacks* – After a while the system, like any other involving machinery, can become monotonous, although exercises can be varied and made more difficult as you become more proficient. Unlike weight training, which is confined to gym equipment, there are a wide range of different exercises that can be added to the basic Pilates routine. These can tax and test your strength, balance, flexibility and co-ordination, which may prove extremely challenging to anybody who sticks with the system. These exercises offer no aerobic work-out, so you should supplement them with another more vigorous activity such as running, swimming or dancing.

### Bouncing

This involves carrying out a variety of skipping, jogging, jumping and kicking movements on a mini-trampoline or bouncer. Bouncing offers a simple form of low impact aerobics which doesn't jar or jolt the spine, knees or ankles as much as jogging.

*Time involved* – You should aim for a daily schedule of at least ten minutes but preferably 20 of intensive activity.

*Weight-loss/body shaping benefits* – If carried out for long periods you can raise the heart rate and increase oxygen intake. However, Dr Kenneth Cooper emphasises that bouncing does not offer an aerobic training effect on a par with cycling, swimming or jogging. Use hand weights or dumb-bells for a tougher work-out, incorporate a skipping rope into your routine or strap ankle weights on while jogging or kicking to increase oxygen consumption. Body shaping potential is very minimal, although bouncing vigorously can strengthen and tighten leg muscles, depending on which leg movements you do.

*Is it right for you?* – It is if you want to exercise at home and need a simple system to do as and when you want. Bouncing is fun, but hardly likely to tax your skill and extend physical prowess. This is a good way of gently breaking yourself into a more demanding aerobic routine if you are very unfit.

*Drawbacks* – Bouncing can become monotonous after the initial novelty and fun wears off. The range of possible movements is limited, and having to stick to one circumscribed area when jogging on the spot is dull and physically restricting.

## Body awareness and conditioning systems (Medau/Mensendieck/Feldenkrais/ The Alexander Technique/Yoga/T'ai Chi)

These are non-violent methods of body conditioning with maximum emphasis on stretching, postural alignment and natural integrated movement to release tension and improve bodily co-ordination and control. Some techniques, like the Alexander Technique, encourage the individual to 'unlearn' incorrect sitting, standing, lying, walking patterns, while others like yoga, T'ai Chi and Feldenkrais, encourage mental and physical harmony.

*Time involved* – Twice or three times weekly hour-long sessions, although yoga asanas (postures) should be performed daily or every other day for 25 to 45 minutes. Consult a trained teacher to learn how to do the exercises correctly. Later you can practice at home with a book for guidance.

*Weight-loss/body shaping benefits* – Unlike cruder 'slam-bang' keep fit exercises, all these systems encourage a greater awareness and sensitivity to how the body works and how to use it properly. Movements are never forced or violent. The goal is usually for each individual to develop his or her naturally integrated and spontaneous patterns and styles of movement, with emphasis on mental and physical co-ordination. The aim is also to overcome bad habits that may have developed as a result of injury, illness, muscular tension or occupation. As the tendency to sag, slouch and hunch parts of the body diminishes and you learn how to hold the body gracefully and correctly, you may also begin to look slimmer and fitter. The ability to relax the body, overcome tension and move in a freer, more co-ordinated way using economical movements, are principal benefits.

Yoga stretches all the muscles, flexes the joints and strengthens the body generally. The Mensendieck exercises can be used remedially after injury or illness and to strengthen the back and tummy; they are also ideal for anyone who is overweight or unfit. The Alexander Technique can help to eliminate aches and ailments associated with tension and incorrect posture. Medau is a creative form of exercise, much of it quite vigorous and especially designed for women, which works the entire body without risk of strain, encouraging grace, agility and strength.

The body shaping potential of all of these systems is fairly modest when compared to dance/calisthenics/weight training/ Pilates. None of the systems will help you burn up extra Calories (kilojoules) and lose weight but, by improving posture and the way you use the body, they can eventually make the body appear straighter, taller and therefore slimmer.

*Is it right for you?* – It is if you are either very unfit, overweight, suffer from faulty posture, injury, a weak back, or simply want to become more tuned-in to the subtler levels of body movement – including breathing, posture, physical sensations. If you are aiming for all-round fitness, use one of these methods to complement a more vigorous form of exercise like jogging and/or weight training.

*Drawbacks* – These include the cost of visiting a class or teacher or the risk of getting it wrong if you work at home alone, although the exercises are safe and you cannot injure yourself. None of these systems may appeal to anyone who is very sporty and action-orientated and likes to sweat a lot. Nor do they produce rapid and visible results, either in fitness levels or improved body shape.

# – 6 –
# *Alternatives*

The growing popularity of alternative medicine reflects our increasing awareness of the closely related functions of mind and body. Treating psyche and soma (body) together, as one single, closeknit and interdependent unit lies at the route of all 'holistic' healthcare. The emphasis is on preventing illness and, where possible, alleviating or removing the underlying cause of health problems, rather than opting for short-term symptomatic treatment.

Consulting a homeopath, naturopath or acupuncturist for a health problem unconnected with slimming, may well result, quite coincidentally, in weight-loss. Almost all natural healing methods such as naturopathy, herbalism and acupuncture are based on the principles of healthy, well-balanced nutrition. While helping you to change your eating habits by eliminating fattening junk foods in favour of more nutritious and often low Calorie (kilojoule) wholefoods, fruit and vegetables, an alternative practitioner could certainly help you to lose weight as an inevitable concomitant to improved health.

In general, however, few alternative therapists are experts on slimming. They operate on the principle of healthy, balanced nutrition which, by its very nature, tends to be non-fattening. Acupuncturists, on the other hand, report considerable success in the treatment of a variety of bad habits and addictions, including the addiction to food.

**Acupuncture**

No one knows exactly how or why acupuncture works in alleviating pain or curing addiction, although there are a number of theories. The most recent explanation put forward by medical doctors who also practice acupuncture, is that inserting needles into certain acupressure points may trigger the release of powerful, morphine-like chemicals known as endorphins. The body manufactures these endorphins automatically in response to stress, pain, injury. Acupuncture is also believed to stimulate the secretion of anti-inflammatory hormones like cortisone, produced by the body to speed healing. Other researchers speculate that acupuncture may work by triggering electrical impulses between nerve cells, thereby helping to elevate pain thresholds.

That acupuncture works in many cases to overcome problems of smoking, over-eating and serious drug addiction cannot be denied. Traditional acupuncture has been used successfully to treat heroin and methadone addicts. Neuro-electric therapy, the much-publicised drug therapy undergone by Boy George and other pop musicians in past years, is simply a more sophisticated electronic technique used to stimulate or sedate the body's acupuncture points.

Acupuncture alone does not, of course, make you give up a habit – whether it is smoking, over-eating or hard drugs. Its value, in any form of detoxification therapy, lies in alleviating or eliminating the often highly distressing and unpleasant physical and psychological side-effects. These often occur when coming off drugs, cigarettes – or going on a diet.

*Strengthening defences*

By strengthening the body's organs, in particular the liver and kidneys, and stimulating the systems associated with digestion and elimination, acupuncture may help the body to re-adjust more quickly and smoothly to changes in diet and lower Calorie (kilojoule) intake. Because acupuncture often helps to relax mind, body and increase energy, the tiredness, dizziness, headaches and irritability experienced by many dieters when cutting Calories (kilojoules) often respond to a series of regular treatments. Weight-gain due to fluid retention may also respond to acupuncture, which encourages the kidneys and lymphatic systems to eliminate surplus fluid more efficiently.

Many acupuncturists emphasise that treatment to help dieters overcome the desire to over-eat or eliminate side-effects of dieting may not have immediate effects. Six to ten treatments of 20 minutes to half an hour may be needed, once or twice weekly to obtain results. Needles are usually inserted into the foot, leg, hand and perhaps the ear, on points related to stomach, liver, kidneys, intestines. These may be left in place for up to 30 minutes and stimulated with a mild electronic charge, or twiddled by hand. The stomach point is often sedated in order to control hunger and ensure correct digestion. Activating the liver point may help to eliminate headaches or migraine associated with dieting.

*Auriculotherapy*

The ear contains a particularly dense concentration of acupuncture points linked to many different parts of the body. In recent years, certain therapists specialising in the treatment of drug addiction, weight problems and smoking, have concentrated on using a simple, often very effective 'short cut' to obtain speedy results. A staple or stud, rather like a small ear-ring, is inserted into a point on the ear-lobe. This point corresponds to the body's hunger reflex point, which is believed to control appetite. The staple is left in the ear for a period of two or three weeks. During this time the wearer can twiddle or press it whenever he or she feels hungry or develops a particularly strong craving for fattening or prohibited foods.

It is impossible to ascertain who will or will not benefit from auriculotherapy for the treatment of weight-loss. Although some acupuncturists report a 50 to 75 per cent success rate in helping people to stop smoking, the figures are certainly lower and less quantifiable when it comes to weight-loss. Some dieters report excellent, long-lasting results, others maintain that auriculotherapy, whether carried out at regular acupuncture sessions, or as a form of self-help where the ear is pegged for weeks at a time, has little or no effect at all.

*Acupuncture: help not cure*
The problem is that, although acupuncture of any sort can help to calm the nervous system and reduce unpleasant withdrawal symptoms associated with dieting, it cannot control the conditioned responses and reflexes often characteristic of over-eating. While acupuncture can reduce the bodily urge to over-eat, it does less to control the underlying emotional drive. This method may work better for people who find that hunger pangs and cravings make it impossible to stick to a diet than for those who eat because they are bored, lonely or depressed.

Not all acupuncturists offer auriculotherapy as a weight-loss treatment on its own. Many of the more traditional practitioners use auriculotherapy only as a back-up to bodily acupuncture, and prefer to treat the body as a whole. The more traditional the acupuncturist's approach the more likely he is to concentrate on changing a person's diet and lifestyle in order to improve their general well-being.

Acupuncture generally does not hurt, although some people experience mild and temporary discomfort when the needles are inserted. When consulting an acupuncturist for the first time make sure he or she is properly qualified and uses either disposable needles or else follows strict sterilisation procedures. As with tattooing, ear-piercing and injections, there is a risk of developing infections and viruses including Hepatitis B and Aids as a result of infection from a contaminated needle.

*Behavioural therapy*

Nowhere is the holistic ethos and recognition of mind-body synergy more pronouced than in modern psychotherapeutic techniques. Therapists are using these nowadays with increasing success to treat eating disorders which range from compulsive bingeing and over-eating to anorexia nervosa. The relationship between the emotions and our need and tendency to over-eat is a highly complex one. It is often closely related to other inner conflicts related to self-images, as well as our attitudes towards our parents and members of the opposite sex. Compulsive over-eating and the tendency to gain excessive weight, or undergo very extreme and rapid weight changes is, according to many psychotherapists and behavioural therapists, often an outward manifestation of very deep inner conflicts and emotional disturbance.

In theory, behavioural therapy or analysis should work well to help people control or change their patterns of eating and relationship to food in general. Like most forms of extreme, supposedly uncontrollable behaviour, over-eating is seen by many therapists as a conditioned response which, because it was learnt, no matter how long ago, can equally well be unlearnt. What is needed is enough time and patience devoted to substituting good, positive habits for bad, negative ones.

**Feminist Psychoanalysis**
**(i.e. The Women's Therapy Centre)**

The most succinct and cogent theory of how the mind/body link manifests itself in eating patterns has been propounded by the psychotherapist Suzie Orbach. She is author of *Fat is a Feminist Issue* and founder of The Women's Therapy Centre in London and the Women's Therapy Institute in New York City. Analysis and therapy are set within a familiar feminist context – the oppression and distorted imagery of women – and are founded on the proposition that compulsive over-eating and persistent weight problems are often symptomatic of deep-rooted, emotional conflict. This idea will come as no surprise to anyone familiar with the rudiments of feminism.

One central premise is that compulsive eating is linked to an unconscious desire to get or stay fat. Recognising this makes it easier to tackle the business of breaking one's addiction to food. Another is that over-eating offers a way of not conforming to the slim, sexy media image of today's ideal woman, a stereotype many women find unreal, frightening and unattainable. Becoming fat is seen as a symbolic rejection of that image and the limitations it imposes on women's role in society. This attitude has its origins in childhood and often develops as an expression of the complex, and sometimes conflict-ridden, relationship between mother and daughter.

Sexual problems often go hand in hand with eating disorders, reflecting many women's inability to feel confident about their sexuality. Thinness is synonymous with sexual desirability, something many women find hard to cope with. Being fat provides a welcome excuse for a women to de-sexualise herself: if relationships with the opposite sex do not succeed it is common, for example, for many to blame their excess weight. The same goes for potential in one's career. 'If only I were thin, my love life and/or career would work out just fine' is a familiar but usually erroneous assumption of many lapsed or would-be dieters. They blame their weight for the problems in their emotional and professional life. In reality, however, such an argument is a perpetual cop-out.

*Eat and keep quiet*

Another issue examined in group therapy is how women often over-eat as a substitute for expressing emotions such as anger, or fully asserting their needs and desires. Compulsive over-eating or bingeing is seen by many psychotherapists as a symbolic way of 'swallowing' or anaesthetising those feelings that women experience as too dangerous to confront or express. Women's inherent, often unrecognised feelings of inadequacy, vulnerability or insecurity about their bodies and sexuality, the doubts about their autonomy and their relationships in general, are issues that come up repeatedly in therapy. So are the perceived images associated with being thin.

Body image and personal esteem are important issues in therapy, and self-acceptance is the key task in group work. Without it, says Suzie Orbach, weight-loss and breaking the addiction to food can only be temporary. Helping women redefine their self-image, eliminating feelings of disgust and self-dislike, is an essential first step to eating less and becoming slim. Why we over-eat as well as why we want to slim make up a conundrum that must first be unravelled before we can lose weight permanently.

*Body awareness*

Visualisation techniques, experiments in body movement and exercises to heighten bodily sensation, self-perception and encourage body awareness are taught for daily practice at home. Experiments with changes of clothing, for instance, wearing 'thin' clothes when still overweight instead of hiding behind drab, shapeless garments, helps further to define the image a woman really wants to project. It also highlights any discrepancy between that and the impression she gives to others. Fat provides a 'buffer' against inner fears and inadequacies and the demands and pressure of daily life, and until she feels safe in her mind and ready to relinquish those layers of protective insulation, it is impossible for a woman to reach a new goal weight and stay thin.

An initial goal of therapy, therefore, is to help give women a greater acceptance of their bodies, whatever the size. Without this, losing weight is a self-defeating exercise because it continues to trigger disturbing feelings. Therapy also consists of in-depth analysis and demystification of the popular myth and symbols synonymous with being fat (i.e. unattractive, mother figure, lazy, lacking in confidence, out of control) and slim (i.e. sexy, athletic, fit, energetic, confident), as perpetuated by the media, advertising, beauty and fashion industries.

*Trusting food*

Re-evaluation of a person's approach to food, observing their present eating habits and then learning how to change them is an important aspect of therapy. Women are encouraged to trust rather than to fear food, to enjoy eating and savour nutritious foods the way 'normal' eaters do and to tune in to stomach hunger as a cue to eating. By learning to gain control over their relationship to food, obsessive over-eaters eventually develop a more discriminating approach to food and a more relaxed attitude towards eating generally. (Even chocolates and ice cream have their place, in moderation.) The idea is to avoid Calorie (kilojoule) counting and making strict rules about 'forbidden foods' versus 'allowed' foods. Neither is a rigid weight reducing diet advocated, because compulsive eating and compulsive dieting are seen as two sides of the same coin. Both are states of being out of control, and dieting, says Orbach, is a stricture imposed from without. Diets don't work, she maintains. In the case of a compulsive eater who is trying to slim, all the compulsiveness previously manifested in over-eating is now invested in a new obsession – staying on the diet.

*Tackling the root cause*

This approach to weight-loss is by no means for everybody. The goal in this type of therapy is not primarily to achieve rapid weight-loss, but to tackle the root emotional causes of over-eating or compulsive binge/diet behaviour. Self-help strategies must also be learnt, to tackle both the cause as well as the actual over-eating.

The method is more likely to prove helpful for those women who have tried unsuccessfully to diet for many years, and for those who regularly gain and then lose large amounts of weight. It is not so helpful for someone who is simply looking for a set of rules and recommendations for fast and effective slimming. Nor will the system appeal to anyone who refutes the basic principles of the women's movement, although therapy is not based on any particularly radical aspects of feminism.

This approach should, however, spark the imagination of anyone seriously committed to changing negative patterns of behaviour, as well as their physical shape. Of all the methods described in this chapter, this appears to be one of the most serious and well-motivated. It treats mind and body as a symbiotic and closely integrated unit.

## Hypnotherapy

This may involve anything from five to 20 hour-long sessions with a qualified hypnotherapist. Audio tapes geared to the specific needs of each patient are made by the therapist and should be used at home to aid relaxation and help control the urge to over-eat. Techniques vary tremendously from therapist to therapist. They include helping patients develop 'aversion' or 'resistance' to fattening foods and teaching relaxation techniques to overcome stress-related eating problems. Hypnotherapy also tackles deep-rooted psychological issues, and changes behavioural patterns that involve food and eating.

Depending on the patient's problem, hypnotherapy may include some or all of these diverse elements.

The drawback of hypnotherapy is that it can prove expensive. A number of sessions are usually recommended to overcome weight problems associated with deep, underlying emotional conflicts.

### Relaxation and calm

Contrary to popular belief, you do not have to be especially 'susceptible' to hypnosis. For many people, the experience of being under hypnosis is no more dramatic than attaining a state of deep physical relaxation, matched by a state of relative mental calm. This relaxed state is, according to therapists, sufficient to promote what they call an 'altered state of consciousness'. In this state, suggestions and instructions from the therapist can register within the subconscious of the listener.

Problems associated with body image, self-confidence, assertiveness and emotions that relate to a person's tendency to over-eat or inability to lose weight permanently, are often discussed in these sessions. Hypnotherapy is often successful in helping those women who have reached the 'plateau' stage of weight-loss, whereby, after initially losing a certain amount, they can go no further.

Achieving an empathetic relationship between therapist and patient is a contributory factor in successful hypnotherapy. Some people may give up after just one or two preliminary sessions, because they cannot develop trust or confidence in the practitioner. In this case it is usually a good idea to try again with another person.

### Achieving the ideal

Visualisation techniques form an integral part of hypnotherapy and patients are usually asked to carry out imaging exercises rather like those used for relaxation or meditation purposes. In these exercises they see themselves in their ideal shape and weight. As this image becomes increasingly imprinted on both the conscious and subconscious, therapists claim that patients automatically begin to remove the obstacles that have prevented them achieving this metamorphosis.

Another aim is to help patients regain their sense of taste and rekindle the sensations of appetite. Many compulsive over-eaters have long lost their sensations because they now only eat compulsively, through habit or emotional need. Suggestion under hypnosis is used to help the individual become aware and appreciate the colours, textures, taste and smells of 'good', non-fattening foods. Similar reverse techniques are used to turn off the desire for sweet, fattening foods. The rituals that surround eating are examined at length in hypnotherapy, and those which militate against successful weight-loss are replaced by others that are more positive.

Perseverence and cooperation on the part of the patient is a prerequisite for successful therapy. It works particularly well for people who need more confidence to help them lose weight. Getting rid of one habit and replacing it with another more positive pattern of behaviour cannot, however, be achieved in a week or a fortnight.

Where hypnotherapy scores over other techniques is in teaching patients to relax and control their desire to over-eat by using simple, auto-suggestion techniques wherever and whenever needed. However, while the success rate for smoking cures via hypnosis is relatively high, the rate for weight-loss is difficult to determine. It is, say therapists, the most difficult problem to treat because we negatively reinforce ourselves two or three times a day when the time comes to eat.

Hypnotherapy is probably a useful technique to try if you have a long-standing weight problem and find it hard to stick to a diet, or stay at your normal weight for long.

**Slimming clubs and groups (e.g. WeightWatchers)**
Slimming groups such as WeightWatchers have been around for over 20 years. Their high membership and burgeoning popularity testify as much to their success rate in helping slimmers attain and maintain a lower weight as to their common-sense approach to weight-loss. Sound psychology, of the straightforward, non-esoteric variety, relaxed camaraderie, and a sensible no-nonsense attitude to food characterise groups like these.

Frequency of meetings varies from group to group, but generally members attend weekly one-and-a-half-hour classes, at which they are discreetly weighed and their current weight-loss recorded. Depending on the area, Weight-Watchers classes, for example, can be small and intimate or made up of 40 or more individuals.

Class 'leaders' are invariably women (men are encouraged to join, but tend to represent a very small percentage of the overall membership) who have succeeded in overcoming their own weight problems. The principle role of the leader is to help motivate members and generally encourage positive attitudes to slimming at every stage of dieting. They help those with problems overcome any obstacles, self-generated or otherwise, that might prevent them getting to grips with their weight problem.

*Tackling temptation*
Behaviour modification, based on simple psychology, is a key element in this type of group work. Members are encouraged to recognise different ways in which they often sabotage their attempts at dieting.

Unlike other group therapy work, whose goal is to delve into deeper psychological conflicts and issues, the focus here is on practical strategies designed to make the work of slimming easier. Real-life situations are dealt with head-on: such specific problems as eating at home where food is an ever-present temptation, eating away from home in restaurants or homes of friends and coping with friends or family members who are uncooperative with regards to slimming. Other typical problems tackled are bad eating habits such as eating too fast or in conjunction with other activities, and overcoming 'comfort eating' or over-eating linked to depression, anger, loneliness or boredom.

Members are generally not encouraged to dwell on their failure at losing weight. Instead, they are positively encouraged. They are given practical and direct help to overcome their frustrations and setbacks, and helped to develop as much commitment as possible to achieving a slimmer figure. Praise, admiration and reassurance amongst members as a whole adds tremendously to the sense of support many derive from attending meetings.

The principles of balanced healthy nutrition, as opposed to fanatical adherence to any one rigid diet, is fundamental to this approach, and emphasis is on helping people change their eating habits for life. Eating sensibly from a wide range of foods and dieting without hunger, deprivation or recourse to unbalanced crash regimes is the nutritional philosophy of these groups. Members are usually warned off pills, injections and other drugs and discouraged from drinking too much alcohol, skipping meals or obsessively counting Calories (kilojoules).

*Cakes not banned*

Infinitely resourceful and imaginative, WeightWatchers, for example, appeals greatly because members are not expected to shun all desserts, cakes and other fattening foods. Instead, they learn to limit their intake and are taught how to prepare tasty and filling alternatives through ingenious use of herbs, spices, fruit, low Calorie (kilojoule) sweetening agents etc.

New members are encouraged to keep a diary or list of foods and are asked to answer a lengthy questionnaire on their health and lifestyle.

Groups such as WeightWatchers will appeal to anyone who finds losing weight a frustrating and lonely business. Such groups provide an ongoing support system made up of other slimmers and slimming 'experts'. Encouragement, handy tips and feedback from other slimmers provide the necessary incentive to persevere and attain a goal weight. If you equate putting on weight with losing face among fellow slimmers – or conversely, losing weight with praise and admiration – you are obviously going to stick to your diet with great dedication.

Members must be prepared to make a commitment in terms of money, time and effort needed to attend regular group meetings. Groups will not appeal to anyone who is not gregarious or prepared to work hard at losing weight. For others, however, the experience of sharing both their triumphs and their setbacks can prove a powerful motivating force. The most obvious drawback, as experienced by many lapsed dieters, is that once they stop attending lectures and lose the support of the group, they are unable to sustain their new eating habits and tend, eventually, to regain weight.

# – 7 –

# *Cosmetic Surgery*

When all else appears to have failed it is tempting to contemplate surgery as a sure – if extreme – bet in acquiring a better body. However, not only is surgery under any circumstances, and for most physical flaws, a very expensive and sometimes risky measure, not to be undertaken lightly, but the limitations of possible physical improvement are also considerable.

Cosmetic surgery is not the answer for anyone with a weight problem. Quite the opposite, since being overweight severely limits the chances of undergoing successful surgery. Being of near-normal weight is chief prerequisite for most cosmetic operations, even a facelift. Most reputable surgeons are loath to operate on the face or body of any prospective patient who is more than a few pounds above normal weight. The reasons for this are self-evident. A skilled surgeon, whether reducing, augmenting or recontouring parts of the body aims for an optimum result based on his patient's present body type and weight, allowing little room for extensive subsequent weight-loss or gain. Indeed, many operations to tighten areas of sagging flesh and loose skin are designed specifically to improve the shape of the body after extreme weight-loss and the inexorable pull of gravity have left the skin and connective tissue slack, sagging and distended. Those people who experience frequent 'Yo-Yo' weight changes are therefore discouraged from undergoing surgery. Those whose weight tends to be steady remain the best candidates.

## Success depends on raw material

A skilled surgeon, relying as much on manual dexterity as a keen eye for aesthetic balance and symmetry, is restricted in the effects he can achieve by the raw material that he works with – in this case the skin and fatty tissue. Therefore, the most successful operations, and those that provide the longest lasting effect, are usually those carried out on women and men of near normal or even underweight, whose skin is still supple and youthfully resilient and who suffer only from localised figure problems. Such problems include heavy sagging breasts or slack abdominal flesh due to hereditary predisposition, ageing or extreme weight-loss.

Because the term 'cosmetic surgery' has a somewhat frivolous ring to it, it is easy to overlook the fact that this is a complex and highly specialised field. It carries the same inherent risks of trauma, discomfort and possible complications as many other more serious forms of surgery. Scare stories filter through about disreputable 'cowboy' surgeons responsible for causing disfigurement, gross scarring, infection or even death as a result of inept surgery. These stories are not merely sensationalist scaremongering, they are generally founded on bitter truths.

## Assessing the risks

The risk of all types of cosmetic surgery cannot be summarily dismissed. Accordingly, doctors always take into account the medical history of anyone about to embark on a surgical method of improvement. Individual skin type, in particular whether it is liable to form raised keloid scars or heal smoothly without complication, greatly influences the results of the trickier operations such as breast or thigh reduction, which involve intensive scarring.

Pre and post operative care of the very highest standard is vital to the safety and success of any cosmetic operation. Bruising, pain and haematoma (extensive bleeding beneath the skin) are predictable by-products, albeit temporary, of certain operations. The risk of infection and worse, damage to a nerve, though rare, may prove more serious and in some cases irreversible.

### Who to go to

But in the end, the success and safety of any cosmetic operation depends almost exclusively on the surgeon's expertise. Finding a skilled and reputable surgeon is no easy matter, especially for those living outside a big city. The problem of access is greater in Britain and in the rest of Europe than in America or Australia, where surgeons maintain a higher profile. The medical climate in general is more attuned to rejuvenation or aesthetic improvement in America and Australia. In Britain the route to a good surgeon still lies via referral from a sympathetic and well-informed GP. If yours is unsympathetic or uncooperative, you are of course fully entitled to seek out one who is more readily disposed to help.

Cosmetic surgery clinics or advisory centres that advertise should in general be avoided. The prices for surgical and clinic fees at these places may be exorbitantly high, consultation is often perfunctory and not necessarily carried out by a doctor, while pre and post operative care may not be the highest standard – and nor may the work of the surgeon. Make sure you check out your surgeon's credentials before seeing him.

Apart from obvious surgical skills and aesthetic sensibilities, you can expect any really top class surgeon to be adept at the fine art of dealing with people's emotions. He should want to discuss sensitive issues such as sex appeal, physical appearance and ageing. The 'why' element of a consultation – a person's motivation in undergoing surgery, is as important as the 'what' aspect of the actual operation and desired outcome. An extensive preliminary consultation between surgeon and patient is essential for both surgeon and prospective patient. It allows the surgeon to familiarise himself with the precise expectations and needs of the patient, while providing the patient with ample opportunity to discover all relevant information about the intended operation.

## What to expect

Cosmetic surgery will inevitably disrupt your lifestyle, well-being and schedule for some weeks, slowing you down and affecting your looks temporarily. Asking a surgeon in advance about what to expect should, however, prepare you for the post-operative recovery period. Unrealistic expectations and demands for the impossible on the part of the patient are, say surgeons, mostly responsible for disappointment and complaints about the degree of improvement ultimately achieved.

Basic surgical techniques have altered little over the past decade, although many minor modifications and refinements instigated by leading surgeons have helped to ensure more natural, and longer-lasting results. Ultimately, however, results do vary inevitably from individual to individual. The final outcome is always determined by such factors as age and body type.

## Breast reduction (Mammaplasty)

Most women's breasts sag with age but chronic backache, neck pain, shoulder tension, faulty posture, dermatitis and weals or ulcers, made by bra straps that cut into the flesh, are some of the woes suffered by women with very heavy outsize breasts. It is a problem that may be hereditary and caused by hormonal imbalance. It can even affect women who are relatively slim. The problem is often compounded by childbirth, breast-feeding, rapid or extreme loss of weight and normal ageing.

Because of the associated discomfort and limitations to lifestyle oversize breasts are regarded more as a health issue and the operation less of a cosmetic procedure than breast augmentation. It is intended to increase comfort and alleviate related health problems. A complicated, major operation, which can take two to four hours and may involve removal of up to two to three pounds (1.3–1.5 kg) of tissue from each breast, removal of surplus breast tissue presents a major challenge to even the most experienced surgeon. The surgeon's goals are to inflict minimal scarring, preserve the sensitivity and erectile functions of the nipples, while sculpting smaller, neater, more symmetrical contours.

Superfluous flesh can be removed by a variety of slightly differing procedures. Care must be taken to remove enough tissue to make the whole operation worthwhile. Although the shape of the breast will become distended as time goes by, due to the pull of gravity, eliminating too little flesh means that sagging and discomfort can recur only months after surgery. Superfluous flesh and skin is generally excised by a crescent-shaped incision made along the fold underneath the breast, and another vertical incision running from the aureola that surrounds the nipple, down to the bottom of the breast. An incision may also be made around the nipple within the surrounding pigmented area, allowing the nipple to be partially detached during surgery and then repositioned during the final stage of surgery. In some cases, where mostly excess skin rather than underlying flesh is removed, the only incision involved may be the one surrounding the aureola. In the case of young women with excessively large breasts that have not yet begun to sag, reduction of tissue can be made via very small incisions within the fold underneath the breast.

*Drawbacks and complications* – Scarring is the most obvious drawback to most forms of breast reduction. Shorter incisions, new refined, invisible or Z-formation stitching techniques, the use of fine adhesive paper tape to flatten the scar during healing, and staples to pull the edges of the tissues together in a neat line without tugging can greatly minimise the extent and unsightliness of scarring, if not eliminate it altogether. There is about a 50/50 chance that a woman who has undergone breast reduction, especially if it involves cutting into the tissues around the nipple, will not be able to breast-feed. A certain partial, though sometimes only temporary, numbness and loss of sensitivity in the nipple itself may also occur as a result of surgery.

This is a very difficult operation and in cases of unacceptable scarring – especially the formation of bunched keloid scars – or unequal breast size, minor, follow-up surgery may be needed about six months later to achieve a more satisfactory and aesthetic effect. Surgeons point out, however, that in the majority of cases a woman's principal criteria in judging the success of the operation are comfort and convenience, not physical attractiveness. Consequently, most express a willingness to alleviate or eliminate their discomfort at the cost of a certain amount of surface scarring or minor distortion.

*What's involved* – One of the most expensive of all surgical procedures, involving about two to five nights in hospital. Breasts are bandaged with gauze and elastic dressings, stitches are removed after ten to 14 days, often in stages, and tape strips applied in their place.

### Stomach reduction (Abdominoplasty)

Often exacerbated through childbirth, massive weight gain and loss, lack of exercise and sloppy posture, a sagging stomach may persist no matter how much weight is lost through dieting. Stomach tightening consists of a relatively straightforward procedure involving a horizontal incision along the pubis, or 'bikini line'. Flesh is pulled back towards the ribs, superfluous tissue trimmed away, and the skin then pulled down, rather like a snug vest, and stitched down again along the bikini line and inside the crease of the groin. The navel is brought through a new opening made in the tightened flesh, leaving a neat line of stitching around the edge.

*Drawbacks and complications* – Surgeons stress that there must be a lot of 'slack' i.e. loose, hanging flesh, to take in, in order to be able to carry out the operation properly in the first place. Abdominoplasty is not an alternative to dieting or a substitute for exercise, rather it is an adjunct to both. It can only be contemplated when weight-loss and exercise have improved the stomach area as far as possible.

Although relatively straightforward, this is a major operation and in some cases as much as 50 per cent of abdominal skin may be removed. Because the tissues are tightly stretched, the patient must lie in bed for at least two to four days following the operation, legs bent to avoid any counter-pull. Movement and posture in the following weeks are normally limited to walking around slowly in a crouched or concave position.

Scarring is neat and may fade. It is usually well hidden by bikini bottoms and briefs. Initial pain or discomfort after the first day or two is replaced by a sensation of numbness which may last for up to six or ten months. As an optional extra to the tummy tuck procedure, some surgeons may simultaneously tighten loose tissue on the inner thigh, since the operation requires the identical incision along the pubis.

Stitches are removed after about two weeks, although tapes may be applied for a subsequent period to prevent stretching of the scars. Activities such as exercise and sex can usually be resumed about four to six weeks after surgery.

*What's involved* – Four to seven nights in hospital and the need to slow down physically for a few weeks.

**Thighs and Bottom**

The notorious pear-shaped British figure, outsize thighs, dropped large buttocks, wads of diet-resistant bulges at the outsides of the thighs which give an unattractive 'riding breech' effect, is an affliction that causes embarrassment and misery to women of all ages. Since such problems are often hereditary in origin (not particularly indigenous to the British and, indeed, very common amongst women of Latin or Jewish descent) weight-loss, exercise and slimming treatments often have no effect in reducing these areas whatsoever. Ageing can make the problem appear worse, as loose skin begins to sag on the inner thigh and flesh becomes dimpled and puckered.

*Not worth the expense*

Only a few surgeons are willing to carry out operations to reduce the volume of thighs and bottom. It is a procedure that is fraught with complications, ultimately offering very unsatisfactory or short-term results. The general consensus, among surgeons and patients who have undergone surgery, is that it simply isn't worth the trauma and expense, except in cases of gross disfigurement. It all looks simple enough on the drawing board, but rarely translates well on living flesh.

In the case of a buttock-lift to reduce heavy, drooping buttocks only, an incision is made in the crease running along from the inner to outer parts of the thigh. A large wedge of skin and fat is removed, which can greatly lift and flatten an area that is overhanging, drooped and fleshy. This, however, has no effect on large, *muscular* buttocks.

In the case of more extensive 'riding breeches', where flab and bulk extend to the inner and outer thighs, the incision is much longer. It begins at the outermost part of the fold beneath the buttocks, extending up towards the hip bone. In such cases the operation becomes a much more major, risky and complicated affair.

By contrast, flabby inner thighs can be tightened relatively simply. An uncomplicated procedure consists of making an incision along groin crease and pulling up, excising and tightening surplus flesh at the top of the thigh.

*Drawbacks and complications* – Extensive and unattractive scarring, much of it visible when wearing a bikini, briefs or swimsuit, makes this type of operation simply a 'trade in' of one type of problem for another.

No surgeon can guarantee how successfully the operation will turn out or how long the results will last. The tissues may begin to spread or droop, pulling the contours out of shape again a few months after the operation. In addition, this type of body sculpting demands craftsmanship and surgical dexterity of the very highest order to avoid asymmetry and lumpiness while achieving just the correct degree of cantilevering and uplift.

*What's involved* – Depending on the degree and area of the body to be reduced, stay in hospital entails complete bed rest for about a week. Once you are up and about it may take up to 14 days before you are allowed to sit in a chair. Uneven, bunched or overgrown scars can be tidied up in a small follow-up operation or six months after the initial procedure.

### Arms (Brachioplasty)
Weight-loss often causes the tissues of the upper arm, especially the underneath part from armpit to elbow, to become distended or wobbly. This can be tightened neatly by making an incision straight along the bone. Because it is a horizontal and not a vertical incision there is little skin tension and the tissues heal quickly. Scars fade well and there is little risk of keloid bunching. The operation to tighten the entire upper arm involves making a long vertical incision underneath, sometimes in a wavy 'Z' or 'W' shape to prevent the scar from shrinking and restricting movement of the arm.

*Drawbacks and complications* – Very few in this case, although there will always be a definite, visible scar running up the length of the arm from the inner side of the elbow to the armpit. Results are invariably successful and the operation may be performed under either a local or general anaesthetic. *What's involved* – About one or two nights in hospital. Recovery time is short. Stitches are removed about one week after surgery, and tapes applied to the wound for about another week. Movement of the arms may be slightly restricted for a few weeks, but discomfort is minimal.

## Liposuction

Conventional surgery – the old 'cut, excise and stitch' procedures traditionally employed by most surgeons to slim down and reshape sagging or outsize parts of the body – is now rapidly being superseded by a controversial and very innovative technique called suction curretage, or liposuction. Instead of being excised, excess flesh is literally vacuumed away from sections of the body, via a small suction tube or cannula, strategically inserted into the tissues.

This procedure is designed to selectively reduce excess localised fat on hips, thighs, bottom, ankles, stomach, chin and upper arm – but only, and here is the drawback, on people who are otherwise slim and relatively young. Fat cells, once loosened and liquidised and siphoned off will not return and the area will not increase in size again unless there is subsequent overall weight gain.

Liposuction is almost certainly bound to be unsuccessful if performed on anyone with a weight problem. Skin above the fatty layer must be relatively taut and elastic, so that once the extra cushioning of fat has been removed, the surface tissue can retract to fit snugly and smoothly over the flat and neater contours. Skin that has become crêpey, thin or distended through age or repeated and extreme weight-loss, will continue to sag loosely after the fatty underlay has been reduced, an effect that can only be removed through surgery. Young women and men in their late teens, twenties and possibly their thirties, with large buttocks, big ankles, isolated wads or rolls of fat around the waist or hips, are the ideal candidates for liposuction.

Depending on its degree and location, all surplus fat may be eliminated in one single operation, or in the case of a more extensive figure problem, over a number of consecutive operations. In theory the procedure allows very specific recontouring, whether the offending area is small and fiddly, as for example around the knees and upper arms, or widespread and expansive. Only surplus flesh that bulges or protrudes is removed, no more no less.

Prior to surgery the surface to be reduced is first mapped out in ink. An injection of the enzyme Hyaluronidase, mixed with a saline solution, causes the fat cells to swell up and liquefy. Under local anaesthetic a narrow suction tube is inserted into the tissues through tiny incisions, some less than 3 cm long, made at carefully calculated points around or along the section being treated. The fat is quickly vacuumed off, about 1 inch (2 cm) beneath the skin's surface, leaving enough fatty underlay to maintain a smooth, even effect. The number of incisions, and where they are made, depends entirely on which part of the body is being re-contoured, the amount of fat to be removed and the shape of a patient's body. The fat is suctioned off in a curved, spoke-like motion, rather than in straight parallel lines. Thus ensures evenness and preserves the natural undulating curve of such parts of the body as the buttocks.

This is a highly skilled procedure that requires as much surgical dexterity and finely tuned judgement as other cosmetic operations. Over-zealous removal of too much fatty tissue can result in a hefty collapse of skin and connective tissue – rather as if an over-stuffed sofa has suddenly had all its stuffing whipped out, eliminating all surface tension and shape. In order to avoid clearly visible and tangible demarcation lines between treated and untreated flesh, removal of fat cells must be graduated, the tissues tapered at the edges to avoid dips and grooves in the upper layers of flesh.

*Drawbacks and complications* – Bearing in mind the list of criteria for successful surgery, it is not so surprising that many earlier reports of the techniques were discouraging to say the least. Risks and drawbacks include high incidence of surface unevenness, the formation of post-operative scar tissue beneath the skin, dimpling or rippling of the tissues and even eventual return of surplus fat. These may perhaps be unnecessarily high risks and drawbacks of an operation that involves both considerable expense and discomfort.

The problem is one of time-lapse, and the laws of nature – in this case involving the fatty tissue itself. No matter how skilfully a surgeon operates, he cannot foresee how the once-tight mass of underlying tissues will redistribute itself to adapt to the new dimensions. It is true that once removed, fat cells do not return, but instead, the remaining tissues often tend to become rearranged into gnarled lumps and bumps. Adequate after-care is an important factor in determining the final outcome of Liposuction. It consists mainly of regular massage treatment to encourage the tissues to settle down smoothly and counteract the formation of dimples, ripples and lumpiness.

### Practice makes it more successful

To be fair, surgeons have now had a few extra years of practice – or should one say, trial and error – to get it right. The procedure is less controversial and purportedly more refined and successful these day than reported five or six years ago. This is probably because doctors are more adept at recognising exactly who they should, and should not, operate on.

Liposuction offers a relatively successful, untraumatic way of eliminating isolated bulges and lumps on an otherwise slim, firm young body. Because no long or multiple incisions are made, there is no scarring. Surgeons can now reduce areas such as knees and ankles, once dismissed as inoperable because of the inability to hide the scar line. The best results so far are reported in the reduction of the hitherto insoluble problem area – thick ankles. Liposuction works well here, as there is relatively little fat to remove and a more neatly circumscribed area to treat. The risk of visible or ugly scarring in all forms of liposuction is relatively small – incisions are short, often hidden in a skin crease, and tend to heal easily and fade well.

Tremendous care must be taken that the veins and blood vessels are not damaged by insertion of the suction tube. However, the more extensive the removal of fat, the longer the operation and the greater the amount of blood lost, with all the attendant risks of major surgery. There is often extensive bruising and considerable discomfort after surgery and in the case of buttock reduction, sitting down may prove uncomfortable for another one to two weeks. Because the underlying tissues may take up to six months to settle and lose their lumpiness, it is impossible to gauge the true degree of success of the operation until some while afterwards.

*What's involved* – Although liposuction is generally performed under a local anaesthetic, the procedure is followed by one to three nights' stay in hospital. During this time tubes are attached to the affected area for 24 hours to drain away the build-up of excess fluid and prevent haematoma (bleeding). Cost varies according to the part of the body treated. In addition, however, you must reckon the extra cost of massage for an extended post-operative period in order to ensure the best results.

# *Index*